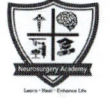 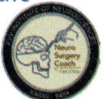
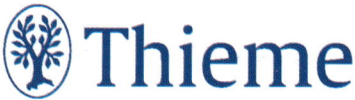

# A Practical Manual for Cisternostomy

## Essentials for Young Neurosurgeons

**Kodeeswaran M., MRCS, MCh (Neurosurgery)**
Neurosurgery Academy and Research Foundation
Professor and Head of the Department
Department of Neurosurgery
Government Kilpauk Medical College
Chennai, Tamil Nadu, India

**J. K. B. C. Parthiban, MCh (Neurosurgery)**
Senior Consultant and Head of Department of Neurosurgery
Kovai Medical Centre and Hospital
Coimbatore, Tamil Nadu, India

**Iype Cherian, MCh (Neurosurgery)**
Neurosurgery Coach
Director, Krishna Vishwa Vidyapeeth Institute of
Neurosciences
Karad, Maharashtra, India

Thieme
Delhi • Stuttgart • New York • Rio de Janeiro

Publishing Director: Ritu Sharma
Development Editor: Dr. Astha Sawhney
Director-Editorial Services:
Rachna Sinha
Project Manager: Ashika Joycell
National Sales Manager:
Bishwajit Kumar Mishra
Managing Director & CEO: Ajit Kohli

Thieme Medical and Scientific
Publishers Private Limited.
A - 12, Second Floor, Sector - 2,
Noida - 201 301,
Uttar Pradesh, India, +911204556600
Email: customerservice@thieme.in
www.thieme.in


Cover design: © Thieme
Cover image source: © Thieme
Page make-up by RECTO Graphics, India


Printed in India by Sanat Printers


5 4 3 2 1


DOI: 10.1055/b000001093


ISBN: 978-81-974758-8-7
Also available as an e-book:
eISBN (PDF): 978-81-967367-6-7
eISBN (epub): 978-81-972990-8-7

**Important note:** Medicine is an ever-changing science undergoing continual development. Research and clinical experience are continually expanding our knowledge, in particular, our knowledge of proper treatment and drug therapy. Insofar as this book mentions any dosage or application, readers may rest assured that the authors, editors, and publishers have made every effort to ensure that such references are in accordance with **the state of knowledge at the time of production of the book.**

Nevertheless, this does not involve, imply, or express any guarantee or responsibility on the part of the publishers in respect to any dosage instructions and forms of applications stated in the book. **Every user is requested to examine carefully** the manufacturers' leaflets accompanying each drug and to check, if necessary, in consultation with a physician or specialist, whether the dosage schedules mentioned therein or the contraindications stated by the manufacturers differ from the statements made in the present book. Such examination is particularly important with drugs that are either rarely used or have been newly released in the market. Every dosage schedule or every form of application used is entirely at the user's own risk and responsibility. The authors and publishers request every user to report to the publishers any discrepancies or inaccuracies noticed. If errors in this work are found after publication, errata will be posted at www.thieme.com on the product description page.

Some of the product names, patents, and registered designs referred to in this book are in fact registered trademarks or proprietary names even though specific reference to this fact is not always made in the text. Therefore, the appearance of a name without designation as proprietary is not to be construed as a representation by the publisher that it is in the public domain.

Thieme addresses people of all gender identities equally. We encourage our authors to use gender-neutral or gender-equal expressions wherever the context allows.

# Contents

# Contents

# Videos

# Foreword

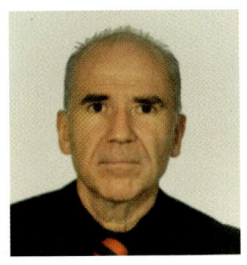

In recent decades, we have seen great advances in management of patients suffering from severe head injury, modern ICP monitoring and control techniques, as well as a better understanding of the value of decompressive craniotomy and surgical indication for brain contusions.

Despite all these advances, results still need to be improved especially in LMICs.

The advent of cisternostomy is another tool in the neurosurgical armamentarium. Using refined techniques, cisternostomy brings to neurosurgery in trauma, the microsurgery and meticulous care of the brain, leading to a thorough, delicate, and useful surgical procedure.

I congratulate Professor Iype Cherian for introducing this concept into neurotraumatology.

**Luis A. B. Borba, MD PhD, IFAANS**
President Elect, WFNS
Professor of Neurosurgery
Federal University of Parana
Curitiba, Parana, Brazil

# Foreword

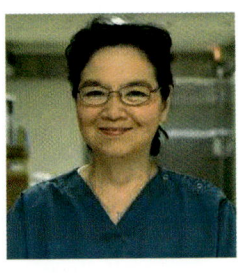

For over the last century, decompressive hemicraniectomy has been the mainstay for head trauma surgery. However, the results have been far from ideal. Professor Iype Cherian started precise microneurosurgery for trauma and the results have been very encouraging as expected when microneurosurgery is employed. Over the last decade and a half, I have been a witness to the acceptance and growth of cisternostomy and I am quite sure it will replace decompressive hemicraniectomy for a lot of indications.

**Yoko Kato, M.D., Ph. D.**
President, Asian Congress of Neurological Surgeons
Chair, Education and Training Committee of the WFNS
First Chair, WFNS Women in Neurosurgery (WIN)
Secretary, WFNS Foundation
Professor, Dept. of Neurosurgery
Fujita Health University, Japan

# Foreword

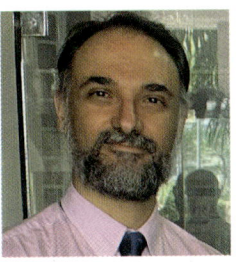

We are living in exciting times, and if you have a true interest in neurotrauma, regardless of your geographical location around the world, you probably have already figured out that the fast pace of change in our theoretical knowledge and surgical capabilities has ignited an irreversible process meant to defy old dogmas and revolutionize standard operating procedures for the management of traumatic brain injury (TBI).

This might possibly be the reason why you decided to approach this topic and read this book on basal cisternostomy (BC). Or, perhaps, you might be skeptical on how such a relatively recent surgical technique could have created so much hype and divergence of opinions across our neurosurgical community. Whatever the reason behind your interest in BC, if you are now reading this book, chances are that you are intellectually honest enough to explore unchartered territories and delve deeper into the roots of the problem.

It is common knowledge that, as in many other aspects of life, progress in surgical practice is made when new incremental advantages are obtained through apparently simple changes; however, this alone is not enough to justify the use of new discoveries. In fact, change usually happens much later when those discoveries are eventually accepted and adopted by the international community. For this, an objective assessment of the journey that has led BC to reach the center stage in the field of neurotrauma is mandatory to assess the roots of the resistance that the proposers of this technique have witnessed so far.

While the mainstay of TBI treatment has always consisted in managing raised intracranial pressure (ICP) via diversion of the impaired cerebrospinal fluid (CSF) dynamics and physical decompression through opening of the dura mater and removal of a large piece of skull, a procedure commonly known as decompressive craniectomy (DC), over time we have acquired a better understanding of the various mechanisms underlying neuroinflammation. This has led few enlightened surgeon-scientists to harness those discoveries and propose the implementation of novel surgical strategies.

Back in 1783, when the Monro-Kelly hypothesis was initially proposed, the intracranial fluids mostly investigated were the blood in the vasculature and the CSF; on the contrary, little was known about intracellular fluid, and even less so about the interstitial fluid (ISF). The discovery of the glymphatic system dates less than two decades ago and the exploration of the mechanisms through which these four fluids are regulated has created the basis for a re-appraisal of the pathophysiology of neurotrauma and neurodegenerative conditions.

In parallel, continuous studies on the anatomy of the brain, and its ventricular systems and basal cisterns have provided a training ground for a new generation of skull base surgeons who developed translatable skills to any other aspect of their neurosurgical practice. Such trend has been recorded all over the world, irrespective of the divisive view assuming the gradient of innovation to be rigidly directed from high- to low- and middle-income countries. As such, neurotrauma, which represents the bulk of neurosurgical practice in most institutions anywhere in the world, particularly in hospitals serving as tertiary major trauma centers, has benefitted from the hands of skills acquired in the anatomical laboratory settings described above. It is therefore unsurprising that BC, initially proposed by Cherian, has found fertile ground for its diffusion from Asia to the rest of the world.

So, what's awaiting us next? Two main issues need to be addressed for the future acceptance of BC as a conventional treatment option in patients with TBI: one is related to the need for clinical evidence and the other is related to the need for appropriate, high-standard, and ubiquitous training. Without further ado, neurosurgeons interested in testing BC must adhere to the ground rules of the scientific method, with the design of international randomized controlled trials meant to test initially the noninferiority of BC to other forms of CSF diversion in the context of surgery for acute subdural hematomas, and eventually the superiority of BC in combination with DC versus DC alone. Only when these steps are accomplished, we will have enough information to possibly consider the idea of a direct comparison between BC and DC as ethically acceptable.

However, for these steps to be accomplished, a standardization of the surgical technique adopted by the various founding fathers of BC will be needed. At present, many variations of the original technique described by Cherian exist, with varying degrees of complexity related to the anterior versus posterior clinoidectomy, and the choice to open the Liliequist's membrane only or to chase a communication between the lamina terminalis and the basal cistern. Steps in this direction have already been taken and personally I am very proud of having contributed to the organization of dissection courses held on the occasion of international neurotrauma conferences supported by national and international neurosurgical societies (see ICRAN 2024).

This book will provide a wonderful resource for any surgeon interested in keeping an open mind and preparing for an argument which will trigger a vivid debate for years to come. The future belongs to the next generation of neurosurgeons, and it might certainly be bright as long as we create the conditions for a respectful international collaboration around the unmet needs of global neurosurgery, with specific attention to the area of neurotrauma, and how to actively contribute to address them.

**Mario Ganau, MD, PhD, MBA, LLM, FEBNS, FRCS(Ed),**
**FFSTEd, FACS**
Nuffield Department of Clinical
Neurosciences, University of Oxford, UK

# The Tree of Life

The Fibonacci series is a fundamental numerical sequence observed ubiquitously in the natural world. The Fibonacci series goes like 1, 2, 3, 5, 8, 13, 21, 34, 55, 89, 144, and so on. The divine proportion, 1.618, derived from the Fibonacci series by dividing any number in the series with the previous one, has been acknowledged for millennia by artists, naturalists, musicians, and astronomers, and is referred to as the divine signature. This pattern of branching can also be identified in the structure of the human brain, mirroring the branching layout of white matter tracts, blood vessels, and notably Virchow-Robin spaces, which play a crucial role in cisternostomy physiology.

# Preface

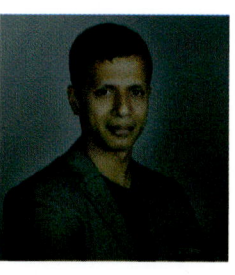

Head trauma is the single most important problem in today's neurosurgical
world. Many lives are lost, while many
stay in a vegetative state, and millions
are spent on this particular issue. Preventive measures
are important, and they are being done all over the world.
However, introduction of microneurosurgery in trauma has
been delayed and this has condemned trauma surgery to be
done by the most junior people without much infrastructure.

Introduction of cisternostomy changes this and while the
results are invariably better as expected with microsurgical
technique, it also gives a different pespective to the way
young neurosurgeons are introduced to microneurosurgical
techniques.

This book follows our 15 years of work during which we
have made a paradigm shift and then swam across the tide to
establish cisternostomy all over the world. The book also dwells
on the aftermath of our thinking process on cisternostomy
where we could explain the role Virchow-Robin spaces in
trauma, cleaning and cooling of the brain, and point toward a
shift in treating neurodegenerative diseases like Alzheimer's.

We believe that it will change the thinking process and
training; and be the beginning of a revolution in neurosurgery.

**Iype Cherian, MCh (Neurosurgery)**

# Acknowledgment

Mr Mario Ganau's contribution has been provided in the context of the Oxford Global Neurosurgery Initiative.

# Contributors

**Ahmed Muthana, MD (Neurosurgery)**
Consultant
Department of Neurosurgery
University of Baghdad
Baghdad, Iraq

**Carlos Salvador Ovalle Torres, MD (Neurosurgery)**
Neurosurgeon
National Autonomous University of Mexico (UNAM)
Certified by the Mexican Council of Neurological Surgery
Fellowship
Autonomous University of Guadalajara (UAG)
Guadalajara, Jalisco, Mexico

**Chirag Hiran, MBBS, MS**
Neurosurgery Academy and Research Foundation
Department of Neurosurgery
Government Kilpauk Medical College
Chennai, Tamil Nadu, India

**Fatimah O. Ahmed, MD (Neurosurgery)**
Consultant
Department of Neurosurgery
Al-Mustansiriyah University College of Medicine
Baghdad, Iraq

**Gidugu Venkata Ramdas, MCh (Neurosurgery) (AIIMS New Delhi)**
Professor and Head of the Department of Neurosurgery
Krishna Vishwa Vidyapeeth
Karad, Maharashtra, India

## Contributors

**Hira Burhan, MBBS**
Research Associate
Department of Neurosciences
Krishna Vishwa Vidyapeeth
Karad, Maharashtra, India

**Ismael Antonio Peralta Baez, MD, MCh**
Consultant
Neurosurgery Department
Hospital Dr. Alejandro Cabral
Dominican Republic

**Iype Cherian, MCh (Neurosurgery)**
Neurosurgery Coach
Director
Krishna Vishwa Vidyapeeth Institute of Neurosciences (KVVINS)
Karad, Maharashtra, India

**J. K. B. C. Parthiban, MCh (Neurosurgery)**
Senior Consultant and Head of Department of Neurosurgery
Kovai Medical Centre and Hospital
Coimbatore, Tamil Nadu, India

**Julio Cesar Perez Cruz, MD (Neurosurgery)**
Main Professor of Academy of Human Anatomy
Higher School of Medicine, National Polytechnic Institute
Bachelor Doctor in Neurosciences
Faculty of Medicine, National Autonomous University of Mexico
Mexico City, Mexico

**Kodeeswaran M., MRCS, MCh (Neurosurgery)**
Neurosurgery Academy and Research Foundation
Professor and Head of the Department
Department of Neurosurgery
Government Kilpauk Medical College
Chennai, Tamil Nadu, India

**Manish Jaiswal, MCh**
Additional Professor
Department of Neurosurgery
King George's Medical University
Lucknow, Uttar Pradesh, India

**Manuel de Jesus Encarnacion Ramirez, MD, MCh**
Senior Resident
Neurosurgery Department
RUDN University
Moscow, Russian Federation

**Naveen Kumar M., MBBS, MS**
Department of Neurosurgery, Government Kilpauk Medical College
Neurosurgery Academy and Research Foundation
Chennai, Tamil Nadu, India

**Osman Elamin, MD (Neurosurgery)**
Consultant
Neurosurgery Department
Jordan Hospital and Medical Center
Amman, Jordan

**Pablo Villanueva, MD (Neurosurgery)**
Neurotrauma Fellow
Department of Neurosciences
Krishna Vishwa Vidyapeeth
Karad, Maharashtra, India

**Priyadharshan K. P., Mch, DrNB (Neurosurgery)**
Neurosurgery Academy and Research Foundation
Assistant Professor
Department of Neurosurgery
Government Kilpauk Medical College
Chennai, Tamil Nadu, India

# Contributors

**Ramesh Chandra V. V., MS, MCh, FRCSed**
Professor and HOD
Department of Neurosurgery
Sri Venkateswara Institute of Medical Sciences (SVIMS)
Tirupati, Andhra Pradesh, India

**Samer S. Hoz, MD (Neurosurgery)**
Research Fellow
Department of Neurosciences
Krishna Vishwa Vidyapeeth
Karad, Maharashtra, India

**Sarita Kumari, MCh, MS, MCh, FRCSed**
Assistant Professor
Department of Neurosurgery
King George's Medical University
Lucknow, Uttar Pradesh, India

**Yonghong Wang, MD, PhD Professor**
Master's Supervisor
Deputy Director of Neurosurgery
Director of Neurological Trauma Ward
Shanxi Bethune Hospital, Shanxi Academy of Medical Sciences
Shanxi, China

# Overview of Traumatic Brain Injury and Need of Cisternostomy in TBI

**1**

*Kodeeswaran M., Priyadharshan K. P., Naveen Kumar M., and Chirag Hiran*

## Introduction

Traumatic brain injury (TBI) presents a significant public health concern on a global scale, demonstrating a consistent epidemiological trend spanning the last three decades. TBI is a notable factor in both mortality and morbidity, particularly in younger individuals. The connection between TBI and both primary and secondary brain damage has been extensively documented. The former, influenced by the intensity of the injury, lacks definitive solutions. Following survival, the secondary damage plays a crucial role, as the absence of effective interventions could lead to complex cascades that worsen cerebral injury.

Despite progress in medical treatments, there is a lack of treatment options to reduce secondary or delayed harm following TBI. Many experimental and clinical studies have thoroughly investigated substances with neuroprotective qualities. However, thus far, all phase III trials have failed to confirm the effectiveness of neuroprotective agents in TBI. Common surgical procedures currently include the placement of external ventricular drains and decompressive craniectomy. Studies suggest that both methods reduce intracranial pressure (ICP), though their impact on outcomes remains uncertain. In light of the challenges in validating neuroprotective agents for TBI, future research may need to explore alternative treatment strategies to effectively address ICP and enhance patient outcomes.

The DECRA study, also known as Decompressive Craniectomy (DC) in Patients with Severe Traumatic Brain Injury, represents the most comprehensive randomized trial dedicated to diffuse TBI.[1] Regrettably, the results of this investigation failed to illustrate the effectiveness of decompressive craniectomy in adult individuals afflicted by TBI. Despite the successful reduction of ICP to atmospheric levels achieved by decompressive hemicraniectomy, it does not address intracerebral pressure, consequently resulting in significant brain swelling and herniation. The exploration of novel approaches such as pharmacological interventions or advanced monitoring techniques could present promising pathways toward effectively managing intracerebral pressure and improving patient outcomes in cases of TBI.

Cisternostomy is an innovative procedure, which was proposed and started by Dr. Iype Cherian from India, that integrates expertise in skull base and microvascular surgery. It has been suggested that during the initial phases of a head trauma, there may be a transfer of cerebrospinal fluid (CSF) from the cerebral cisterns to the brain, resulting in significant brain swelling. By exposing the brain cistern to atmospheric pressure, cisternostomy has been proven to reduce ICP through the redistribution of CSF across the Virchow-Robin (VR) spaces.[2-4]

Nevertheless, it is important to acknowledge that accessing the cisterns in a swollen brain affected by TBI is a complex task that demands a comprehensive understanding of anatomy and substantial surgical expertise.

Its foundation lies in the theory of CSF shift edema, which associates brain injury with elevated pressure within the subarachnoid space resulting from hemorrhage and compromised glymphatic drainage. Initial findings suggest that cisternostomy has the potential to bring about notable enhancements in clinical results, manifesting as decreased mortality rates, shorter durations of stay in the intensive care unit (ICU), and improved scores on the Glasgow outcome scale (GOS). Despite the promise it holds, the integration of cisternostomy has been gradual, primarily due to the considerable learning curve involved and the necessity for proficient microsurgical abilities.[5,6] Research has indicated that cisternostomy, whether performed independently or as a supplementary procedure to DC, may prove more efficacious in managing ICP and minimizing complications when compared to the sole utilization of DC. Nonetheless, the available evidence remains restricted, with the majority of studies being confined to reports from single centers with limited sample sizes. Particularly in low- and middle-income countries (LMICs), where it was initially developed, this procedure has demonstrated potential by providing a cost-effective resolution to the substantial burden of TBI. Although suggestions have been made for cisternostomy to supplant DC due to its reduced morbidity and mortality rates, further investigation is imperative to definitively establish its efficacy and safety.[7] In essence, cisternostomy signifies a noteworthy progression in neurosurgical methodologies for TBI; nevertheless, its widespread acceptance hinges on the availability of more robust clinical data and training initiatives to surmount the technical obstacles.[8]

# Conclusion

Cisternostomy represents an innovative surgical approach for severe TBI, although the concept of cisternal opening is a well-established principle in neurosurgical practice. Currently, the technique can be viewed as a supplementary surgical maneuver in conjunction with decompressive craniectomy. However, upon definitive confirmation of its efficacy, it possesses the potential to supplant decompressive craniectomy in the management of severe TBI. Innovative surgical techniques like cisternostomy hold promise for advancing the management of severe traumatic brain injuries beyond traditional practices. Exploring novel surgical methods such as cisternostomy could revolutionize the treatment of severe traumatic brain injuries by expanding beyond conventional approaches.

# References

1.  Chi JH. Craniectomy for traumatic brain injury: results from the DECRA trial. Neurosurgery 2011;68(6):N19–20
2.  Cherian I, Bernardo A, Grasso G. Cisternostomy for traumatic brain injury: pathophysiologic mechanisms and surgical technical notes. World Neurosurg 2016;89:51–57
3.  Wu J, Zhou A, Huang Z, Li L, Bai H. A facile method to prepare three-dimensional $Fe_2O_3$/graphene composites as the electrode materials for supercapacitors. Chin J Chem 2016;34(1):67–72, Cover Picture
4.  Grasso G. Surgical treatment for traumatic brain injury: is it time for reappraisal? World Neurosurg 2015;84(2):594
5.  Hoz SS, Alramadan AH, Hadi AQ, Moscote Salazar LR. Cisternostomy in neurosurgery: a new proposed general classification based on mechanism and indications of the cisternostomy proper. J Neurosci Rural Pract 2018;9(4): 650–652

6. Servadei F, Kolias A, Kirollos R, Khan T, Hutchinson P. Cisternostomy for traumatic brain injury—rigorous evaluation is necessary. Acta Neurochir (Wien) 2020;162(3):481–483

7. Kanmounye US. The rise of inflow cisternostomy in resource-limited settings: rationale, limitations, and future challenges. Emerg Med Int 2021;2021:6630050

8. Kyaruzi VM, jean de Dieu TM, David S, et al. Comparing the therapeutic effects of cisternostomy versus decompressive craniectomy in the management of traumatic brain injury—systematic review and meta-analysis protocol. medRxiv 2023. doi: 10.1101/2023.03.06.23286840

# History and Evolution of Cisternostomy

**2**

*Iype Cherian*

## Introduction

In this chapter, we talk about the discovery and evolution of cisternostomy.

## Serendipitous Discovery of Cisternostomy

Circa 2007, the author was working at Aleppey Medical College as a lecturer in neurosurgery. The place was close to his home and being near the sea was something he loved.

The Neurosurgery Department at Christian Medical College, Vellore, where he was doing his residency at that time, was one of the best in the subcontinent and the discipline and the knowledge that Vellore imparted have stood like a pillar in his career.

The author had seen and done many decompressive hemicraniectomies for trauma during his stint in Vellore. It is the most desperate and the easiest of surgeries for the largest volume of neurosurgical cases. It presented no surgical challenges for the young neurosurgeon who wanted to embark on a journey of improving his skills, along with no hope for the patient.

The lectures on the "Technique of Decompressive Hemicraniectomy" was the only time one would actually be convinced that monkeys could do neurosurgery, as their incumbent Chief of Neurosurgical Services at that period Professor Vedantam Rajshekhar always kept reminding them.

It was later in his career that the author found out that decompressive hemicraniectomies for trauma were so difficult to replace owing to exactly this ease of doing it and the lack of need for any infrastructure or special skills for this surgery. Decompressive hemicraniectomy was a 120-year-old procedure, mostly done by junior residents with no microscopes. Any beginner neurosurgeon could always thrive by doing this in any small nursing home.

Many studies done on the efficacy of decompressive hemicraniectomy had come to the conclusion that it was probably only effective in changing the status from death to a vegetative state at best.[1,2]

Any patient who survived the first procedure had to undergo cranioplasty. This was another simple procedure to put the bone back. However, by the time the patient undergoes this second procedure, the side of the decompressive hemicraniectomy brain often looks hollowed out with actual brain tissue loss of up to 70%. This is because of the brain tissue herniating into the decompressive craniectomy (DC) site and sustaining severe stretch damage to tracts and cortex.

So, with this background, in 2007 in Alleppey, while the author was working as a lecturer in neurosurgery, the alleged story goes that he had mistook a case of severe head injury as an Acom aneurysm and proceeded to do everything that he would do for an aneurysm, without obviously finding the aneurysm. By the time he figured this out, the cisterns were open as was the routine for any aneurysm surgery, and the brain was quite lax.

Rather than getting upset about the mix up, he observed that the head injury and the aneurysmal subarachnoid hemorrhage looked very similar, and both would become lax once you proceeded to open the cisterns. For this case, they did not put the bone flap back, even though the brain was quite lax. Generations of teaching DC was deeply ingrained into their minds. The next day, the patient was almost ready to be extubated and that night he decided to question the Monro Kellie Doctrine, and a hundred years of "fear of the malignant brain swelling," the routine practice of not using the microscope in trauma, and the continuing decompressions through four generations of neurosurgeons.

They started opening the cisterns along with doing decompressive hemicraniectomy and very soon they realized that once the anterior and posterior cisterns (membrane of Liliequist) are opened and if a drain is put in for 5 days to drain the cerebrospinal fluid (CSF), the bone can be kept back. Keeping the bone back was way better for the patient than combining cisternostomy with DC. They started doing isolated cisternostomy and started better selection criteria as well as started improving the surgical technique.[3]

However, when they started to present this and publish this, they faced sheer resistance and ridicule just like any new procedure which made people insecure. Till then trauma surgeons hardly needed to operate, and most of them were excellent writers. Their presentations were mostly hovering on the hopeless scenario in decompression done by their junior residents, and the whole theme of head injuries was slowly moving toward a nonsurgical management with so-called intensivists calling the shots.[4]

When cisternostomy arrived, these fantastic writer-presenters had to become fantastic skull base surgeons, and this was not an easy overnight transition. The easier path was to nonsense it for lack of evidence and lack of scientific methodology, which was their expertise. Fortunately, good skull base surgeons from India and all over the world took notice and in 15 years, the surgery found its way all over the world with numerous publications and two randomized controlled trials to date.[5] Of particular note would be Professor Ghuo Yi and Professor Wang from China,[6] Professor Roy Daniel and Professor Lorenzo Giammattei from Switzerland,[7] Professor Antonio Bernardo from the US, Professor Parthiban,[8] who was instrumental in convincing others with his simple and elegant ways of explanation and surgical technique, Professor Ramesh Chandra,[9] Professor Manish and Professor V. D. Sinha, Professor Sumit Sinha, Professor Deepak Gupta from India, and more than 40 of the author's fellows from all over the world.

Over the last decade and a half, they learned a lot and understood that perioperative care in the ICU was as important as the procedure itself and a combined work of the surgeons and the medical management was the best of both worlds. They have made sure that they have Neurocritical Care Department with them who helped them to manage the odds better in both the operating room and the ICU from then on.

After conducting a complete session on cisternostomy in WFNS Beijing in 2019 and after leading this year's (2024) World Neurotrauma Congress workshop on Cisternostomy, and after hearing countless surgeons' accounts of saving meaningful lives with cisternostomy from all over the world, the author has the satisfaction of changing the management of the largest caseload (head trauma) of neurosurgeons all over the world with the added benefit that neurosurgery residents are becoming better surgeons with cisternal surgery, as Yasargil would have envisioned.

The author met Professor Gazi Yasargil in 2012 in Turkey. He had been presented the Tetsuo Kano prize for the best presentation (I talked on cisternostomy) in Asian Congress. The author met him again in 2018 while in Istanbul for an invited lecture on cisternostomy with his friend, philosopher, and guide, Juha Hernesniemi. The author remembers Professor Yasargil telling him that he should get a Nobel for cisternostomy after listening to their journey on this. This would certainly count as one of the proudest moments of the author's career. Nobel or not, he certainly cherishes all the efforts, criticism, and the subsequent recognition for changing the course for head injuries all over the world forever.

## Philosophy of Cisternostomy and the Line of Thinking from Cisternostomy to the Cleaning and Cooling

**After the serendipitous discovery of cisternostomy, here the author describes what happened next in their journey...**

A few questions that the author used to ask himself before he understood more about cisternostomy were:

*Where does all the CSF in the basal cisterns go to in severe head trauma (when the scan shows literally no cisterns at all)?*
*Why is the CSF changed three times in a day?*

After cisternostomy started working, the author started the quest to find out how it worked. He hypothesized that the CSF in the basal cisterns was being displaced into the brain. This explained the very high pressure within the brain and the absence of CSF within the cisterns in scans and surgery. There was just blood in the cisterns. After studying the anatomy and physiology of how CSF is secreted and how it is absorbed, he realized that the cisternal CSF is going into an extensive network of Virchow Robin spaces present around the vessels.

CSF is not compressible and there is 120 mL of CSF in the basal cisterns. Most neurosurgeons believed that in severe head injury, the cisterns are compressed (with the CSF within it) or that the CSF displaced into the spinal subarachnoid compartment. While the first assumption would be completely against the basic laws of physics, the second would cause very high pressures in the spinal subarachnoid compartment. In fact, if this was so, decompressive hemicraniectomy would never have started.

Theodore Kocher[10] did lumbar puncture pressure studies, and he did not find raised ICP. However, since there were clinical signs of raised ICP, he wrongly concluded that decompression should be done.

In trauma, as there was subarachnoid bleeding, this would raise the pressure within the cisterns. The blood was a newcomer into the cisterns and the pressure at which the capillaries within the cisterns bleed would raise the pressure to 40 mmHg and above. Since the red blood cells would not be able to shift into the Virchow Robin spaces, it was the CSF that would shift into the extensive network of Virchow Robin spaces till the cisterns are full of blood and the Virchow Robin spaces across the brain is full of CSF. This would tremendously raise the pressure within the brain parenchyma and the cerebral perfusion pressure would be soon at risk, causing secondary ischemic injuries and starting a vicious cycle.[11] This theory was making sense and the author started talking about it from 2009 onwards.

Decompressive hemicraniectomy just causes a herniation of the brain equivalent to the amount of CSF forced in from the cisterns.

After the author figured out that the "CSF shift edema" was responsible for the high intraparenchymal pressure and absence of cisterns on the scan, he wanted to know why physiological pathways for the CSF from the cisterns into the brain exist.

As he researched more, he understood that the CSF was going in through the Virchow Robin spaces which was surrounding the blood vessels traversing from the cisterns into the brain, and once he figured out about the Archimedes screw principle in Tours, France while visiting Leonardo DaVinci's resting place, he knew this was how the CSF was driven in. The pulsations of the vessels drove the CSF in the Virchow Robin spaces surrounding the vessels.[12]

The proximity of the cisterns to nasal sinuses and the sella got him thinking again. With his interest in automobiles and physics, it was easy to see that the sinuses are the radiators in the brain. He hypothesized that, while breathing happens, the air enters the sinuses through very small entry pores into the sinuses, which would accelerate the air velocity (Bernoulli's principle) and would result in evaporation of the water content in the sinus mucosa and cooling of this area. More than 500 mL of water is evaporated every day for this purpose.

The sinuses cool the surrounding areas, and it is no coincidence that the largest CSF cistern is right in the middle of the sinuses. He proposed that this will cool the CSF and this cooled CSF was being used to cool the rest of the brain as it is pumped into the Virchow Robin spaces using the pulsatility of the vessels.[13]

The author also believes that the pituitary needs to be cooled for some reason and this is why it has been placed in the sella, in the middle of all those sinuses which are the air conditioning system for the brain. Maybe losing the nasal mucosa in the sinuses is not a great result for the pituitary gland and we have started conserving the mucosa for transnasal transsphenoidal surgeries as much as possible.

The author thinks that many degenerative diseases may be caused, or are aggravated, by decreased cooling of the CNS and Uhthoff's symptoms in multiple sclerosis is just one example. From figuring out the anatomy and physiology of how cisternostomy works to hypothesizing how the brain cools and cleans was a journey that the author enjoyed thoroughly.

## Acknowledgment

Dr Margarita Beltran and Dr Hira Burhan have been helpful in discussing and researching and writing these ideas up and publishing them. Without them, these ideas would have remained in the back of the author's mind without ever being published, and he owes a great deal of gratitude to both.

## References

1.  Cooper DJ, Rosenfeld JV, Murray L, et al; DECRA Trial Investigators; Australian and New Zealand Intensive Care Society Clinical Trials Group. Decompressive craniectomy in diffuse traumatic brain injury. N Engl J Med 2011;364(16):1493–1502
2.  Hutchinson PJ, Kolias AG, Timofeev IS, et al; RESCUEicp Trial Collaborators. Trial of decompressive craniectomy for traumatic intracranial hypertension. N Engl J Med 2016;375(12): 1119–1130
3.  Cherian I, Yi G, Munakomi S. Cisternostomy: replacing the age old decompressive hemicraniectomy? Asian J Neurosurg 2013;8(3):132–138
4.  Servadei F, Kolias A, Kirollos R, Khan T, Hutchinson P. Cisternostomy for traumatic brain injury—rigorous evaluation is necessary. Acta Neurochir (Wien) 2020;162(3):481–483
5.  Cherian I, Bernardo A, Grasso G. Cisternostomy for traumatic brain injury: pathophysiologic mechanisms and surgical technical notes. World Neurosurg 2016;89:51–57
6.  Wang Y, Liang L, Sun J, et al. Effect of cisternostomy on prognosis of patients with traumatic brain injury. Chinese Journal of Trauma 2019;(12):389–393

7.  Giammattei L, Messerer M, Oddo M, Borsotti F, Levivier M, Daniel RT. Cisternostomy for refractory posttraumatic intracranial hypertension. World Neurosurg 2018;109:460–463

8.  Parthiban JKBC, Sundaramahalingam S, Rao JB, et al. Basal cisternostomy—a microsurgical cerebro spinal fluid let out procedure and treatment option in the management of traumatic brain injury. Analysis of 40 consecutive head injury patients operated with and without bone flap replacement following cisternostomy in a tertiary care centre in India. Neurol India 2021;69(2):328–333

9.  Chandra VVR, Mowliswara Prasad BC, Banavath HN, Chandrasekhar Reddy K. Cisternostomy versus decompressive craniectomy for the management of traumatic brain injury: a randomized controlled trial. World Neurosurg 2022;162: e58–e64

10. Rossini Z, Nicolosi F, Kolias AG, Hutchinson PJ, De Sanctis P, Servadei F. The History of Decompressive Craniectomy in Traumatic Brain Injury. Front Neurol. 2019;10:458.

11. Cherian I, Beltran M, Landi A, Alafaci C, Torregrossa F, Grasso G. Introducing the concept of "CSF-shift edema" in traumatic brain injury. J Neurosci Res 2018;96(4):744–752

12. Cherian I, Beltran M. Unified physical theory for CSF circulation, cooling and cleaning of the brain, sleep, and head injuries in degenerative cognitive disorders. In: Opris I, Casanova MF, eds. The Physics of the Mind and Brain Disorders. Springer Series in Cognitive and Neural Systems. Springer Cham; 2017:773–783. Accessed May 19, 2024 at: https://ouci.dntb.gov.ua/en/works/4KjJE6J7/

13. Burhan H, Cherian I. Brain Cooling and Cleaning: A New Perspective in Cerebrospinal Fluid (CSF) Dynamics. In: Ambrosi PB, Ahmad R, Abdullahi A, Agrawal A, eds. New Insight into Cerebrovascular Diseases—An Updated Comprehensive Review. www.intechopen.com. Published February 21, 2020. Accessed at: https://www.intechopen.com/chapters/71184

# Anatomy and Understanding of the Cisterns: Microsurgical Anatomy of the Basal Cisterns and Surgical Landmarks for Cisternostomy

**3**

*Pablo Villanueva, Carlos Salvador Ovalle Torres, and Julio César Pérez Cruz*

## Introduction

Arachnoid cisterns are crucial in neurological surgical procedures. They act as surgical corridors, allowing surgeons to move between different structures and cavities and access the various vessels and nerves within each cistern. This system is invaluable for reaching various types of lesions in the brain, including tumors, vascular malformations, aneurysms and more.

As we will see later in this chapter, the cisterns are also essential for surgery on severe traumatic brain injury, and are useful in any pathology that presents with diffuse cerebral edema. It will aim to provide clear anatomical guidance about the main relevant basal cisterns involved in the cisternostomy procedure. It begins with a definition of what a cistern is, and then goes on to simplify the anatomical details. It also offers tables and graphic aids for better understanding.

A cranial arachnoid cistern is defined as the space between the two known layers of soft meninx, arachnoid and pia mater, forming a special cavity bigger than the rest of the subarachnoid space that covers the cortex. This is larger than the subarachnoid space that exists between adjacent cerebral gyri of the cortex. It can contain vascular and nervous structures. The arachnoid layer covers the entire surface of the brain without penetrating deep landmarks, adhering closely to the dura surface and bridging significant distances. The internal layer, pia mater, penetrates every single fissure, following vessels up to the microcirculation level. It marks a three-dimensional tube around them, which is named the perivascular space of Virchow-Robin.[1-3]

There is also a spinal subarachnoid space, which is a major component of this group. However, its specific anatomical details will not be discussed in this chapter, which is focused on the cisternostomy procedure.[4]

The concept of "basal cisterns" refers to the cisterns located at the central space between the basal aspect of the brain and the skull base central region of the middle fossa and its transition to the posterior fossa. These cisterns communicate the supratentorial and infratentorial subarachnoid spaces, as well as left and right side of the brain.

The named concept has been described by many authors since the 17th century (Ruysch et al[5]). They have adapted, transformed, and classified these names in different ways, but the first complete description, given by Professor Yasargil[6] in the mid-1970s, is the most widely used. We have followed the FIPAT/IFAA chapter for neuroscience[7] regulations (terms number 285 to 316).[8–10]

For a general overview of the cisterns, please refer to **Table 3.1** and **Table 3.2**. Additionally, **Fig. 3.1** provides a simplified representation of the general flow of the cerebrospinal fluid (CSF) and a schematic of the cisterns.

The cisternal spaces are filled with CSF and are traversed by structural elements (i.e., a nerve or a vessel). Together, the cisternal spaces act as a reservoir, forming part of the total intracranial volume.

Approximately 125 mL corresponds to cisternal CSF (75% spinal/25% cranial)[11] and the subarachnoid space. The remaining 25 mL is ventricular CSF, giving a total volume of 150 mL in the adult.[12] The cisternal and ventricular systems are only connected via the lateral aperture of the fourth ventricle (foramen of Luschka) to the cerebellopontine cistern and the median aperture of the fourth ventricle (foramen of Magendie) to the posterior cerebellomedullary cistern or cisterna magna. These connections have substantial differences in their macroscopic and microscopic composition and properties regarding the flow of the CSF **(Fig. 3.1)**. Once in the cisternal space, CSF can move from one compartment to another.

The compartments are separated by an incomplete porous wall with openings of varying sizes.[6,13] Trabecular adhesions between its walls give this space the common name of "subarachnoid" space. The latter is not a minor detail; these adhesions become the main challenge while dissecting a cistern, manipulating its contents or opening a surgical pathway between them.

Detailed microsurgical information will allow the reader to better understand the specific anatomical scenario of a

**Table 3.1**    Cerebral cisterns: names and nomenclatures

| English name | Latin (FIPAT//IFA) | Other names |
|---|---|---|
| Superficial Sylvian | *Cisterna Fassae Leteralis Cerebri* | Frontotemporal lips, Sylvian fissure |
| Deep Medial Sylvian | *Cisterna Vallecula Cerebri* | Sphenoidal compartment of the Sylvian fissure |
| Deep Lateral Sylvian | *Cisterna Fassae Lateralis Cerebri* | Operculoinsular compartment of the deep Sylvian fissure |
| Carotid | *Cisterna Carotica* | |
| Olfactory | *Cisterna Olfactoria* | |
| Lamina Terminalis | *Cisterna Laminae Terminalis* | |
| Chiasmatic | *Cisterna Chiasmatica* | |
| Interpeduncular | *Cisterna Interpeduncularis* | Intercrural |
| Crural* | ***(Not appearing at FIPAT/ IFA)*** | Lateral Mesencephalic |
| Ambient | *Cisterna Ambiens* | Lateral Mesencephalic |
| Prepontine | *Cisterna Prepontina* | |
| Cerebellopontine | *Cisterna Cerebellopontina* | Pontocerebelosa |
| Premedular* | *Cisterna Premedullaris* ***(FIPAT/IFA 2019 revision)*** ***(Nat Appearing at FIPAT/ IFA 2020 revision)*** | |
| Lateral Cerebellomedular | *Cisterna Cerebellomedulloris lateralis* | |
| Posterior Cerebellomedular | *Cisterna Cerebellomedullaris posterior* | Magna |

Note: *IFA/FIPAT has a 2019 publication where **premedular cistern** appears, but it is not present in the 2020 revision. The **crural cistern** did not appear in 2019 nor in 2020 revision.

Source: Reproduced with permission from Surgical Neurology International.[4]

**Table 3.2** Cisternal membranes: basic description

| Membrane name | Approximate insertions* | Main relations |
|---|---|---|
| Sylvian (superficial) | Arachnoid covering cerebral convexity, bridging frontal and temporal lips surface | Between superior temporal gyrus and inferior frontal gyrus; at the anterior 1/3 conforms the Pars Triangularis widening |
| Carotid lateral and medial sheets | Both membranes join and surround the Carotid Artery just before its A1-M1 bifurcation. The space limitated is: lateral carotid surface, optic nerve-chiasm-tract and the 3rd cranial nerve | Chiasmatic and interpeduncularis cisterns are medially/ sphenoidal part of silvian cistern is laterally/olfactory and lamina terminalis cistern, anteriorly/ over the lateral sheet: optico-carotid triangle is identified |
| Liliequist Diencephalic | Dorsum sellae - posterosuperiorly directioned to the Mamilar Bodies | Chiasmatic cistern anteriorly/conforms the interpedunclaris cistern anterior wall—roof |
| Liliequist Mesencephalic | Dorsum sellae - posteroinferiorly directioned to the 3rd nerve emergence at the pontomescencephalic junction. Involves the PCA and SCA surfaces | Crural—Ambiens Cistern at both sides/ prepontine cistern caudally/conforms the interpeduncularis cistern floor |
| IIIrd nerve cuff | Around the IIIrd nerve, apparent origin at the anterior wall of the Mescencephalon | Intersection of the medial sheet carotid— mesenchephalic liliequist—lateral pontomesencephalic and anterior prepontine membranes |

(Continued)

**Table 3.2** (*Continued*)

| Membrane name | Approximate insertions* | Main relations |
|---|---|---|
| Lamina Terminalis | From the anterior white commissure to the optic chiasm superior surface | Conforms the posterior wall of the lamina terminalis cistern and the anterior wall of the 3rd ventricle/membrane anterior and lateral expansions to the frontal lobes rectus gyrus |
| Lamina Terminalis (Lateral expansion) | From the chiasm to the rectus gyrus inferior surface/ascending direction | Conforms an incomplete division from the sylvian and olfactory cisterns |
| Lamina Terminalis (Medial expansion) | From the chiasm to the rectus gyrus medial surfae/horizontal direction | Conforms an incomplete division from the lamina terminalis cistern and the pericallosal cistern |
| Lateral ponto-mesencephalic | From the pontomesencephalic sulcus, sharing insertion with the IIIrd nerve cuff and the mesencephalic liliequist—going laterally—reaches the superior aspect of the cerebellar lobule and some transtentorial trabeculae up to the uncus and parahippocampus | Bridges the space between the brainstem and the cerebellar surface conforming the division between the crural-ambiens from the cerebello pontine cisterns |

(*Continued*)

**Table 3.2** (*Continued*)

| Membrane name | Approximate insertions* | Main relations |
|---|---|---|
| Anterior prepontine | From the IIIrd nerve cuff runs straight downward to the VIth nerve apparent emergence at the pontomedullaris junction | Prepontine cistern between right and left anterior prepontine membranes/conforms the medial wall of the cerebellopontine cistern |
| Lateral pontomedullaris | From the VIth nerve arachnoid cover at the pontomedullaris junction—laterally projected to the IXth nerve arachnoid cover—finally blends wthi the cerebellar surface arachnoid cover/near the midline, this layer gets thicker but with an orifice for vertebrobasilar confluence and passage | Conforms the floor of the prepontine cistern and cerebellopontine cistern, separating them from the premedullaris and lateral cerebellomedullaris, respectively |
| Intracrural | From the Uncus point (1/3 posterior joins 1/3 midportion of the Uncus) and parahippocampal surface to the medial carotid sheet | Separates crural cistern in superior and inferior compartments for AChorA and PComA respectively |

Note: *Arachnoid membranes are variable in location and presence (they might be absent). Nevertheless, the content and related structures are constant, serving as a stable parameter for a proper cistern identification.
Source: Reproduced with permission from Surgical Neurology International.[4]

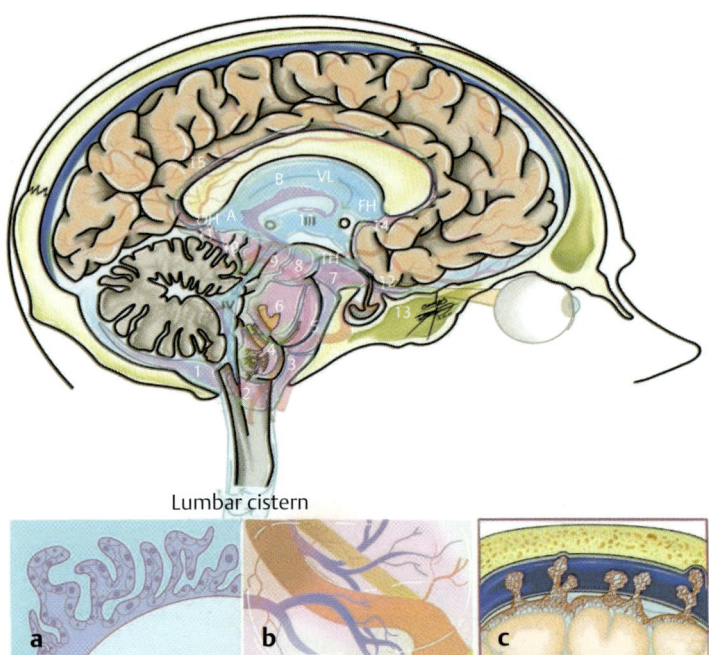

Lumbar cistern

**Fig. 3.1** Schematic diagram of a sagittal view of the production of cerebrospinal fluid and its passage from the ventricular system to the subarachnoid space and the arachnoid cisterns. The listed cisterns are observed: 1. Magna, 2. Lateral cerebellomedullary, 3. Prebulbar/Premedullary, 4. Bulbocerebellar, 5. Prepontine, 6. Pontocerebellar, 7. Interpeduncular, 8. Crural (anterior ambiens), 9. Ambiens (posterior ambiens), 10. Quadrigeminal, 11. Velum interpositum, 12. Chiasmatica, 13. Lamina terminalis, 14. Pericallosa (anterior portion), 15. Pericallosa (posterior portion). A, atrium; B, body of lateral ventricle; FH, front horn; OH, occipital horn; TH, temporary horn; VL, lateral ventricle. **(a)** Approach to the choroid plexus in the floor of the lateral ventricles and roof of the third and fourth ventricles where cerebrospinal fluid is produced. **(b)** Cisternal space filled with cerebrospinal fluid with vascular and nervous contents. **(c)** Arachnoid villi at the level of the convexity of the superior sagittal sinus, where the cerebrospinal fluid is reabsorbed. Used with permission from Dr. Carlos Salvador Ovalle Torres.

cisternostomy procedure. As the main surgical objective is to reach a specific cistern (**Fig. 3.2a, b**) (the upper part of the prepontine cistern or the transition between the interpeduncular cistern and the prepontine cistern),[4] it is imperative to follow a safe route, to get this millimetric-precise destination.

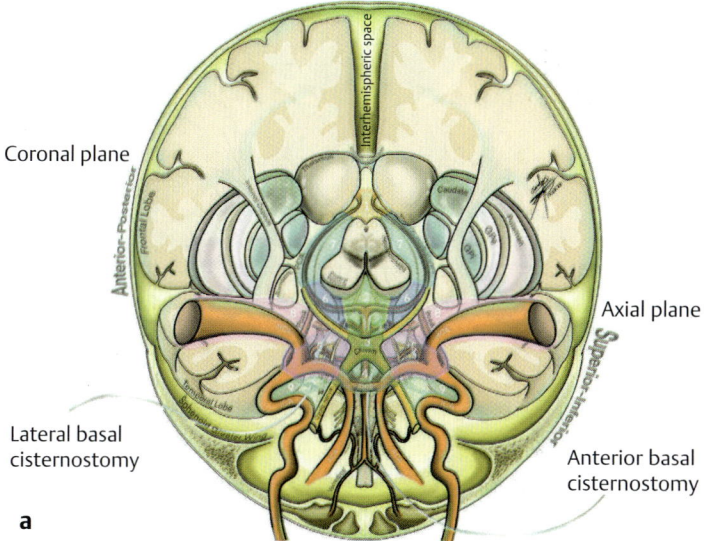

**Fig. 3.2** (**a**) Axial and coronal multiplanar panoramic schematic overview of the anatomy of the skull base, including the main vascular, osseous, and nervous anatomical details as well as the basal cisterns. The route to follow for the lateral basal and anterior basal cisternostomy is shown, with the tip of the catheters in the interpeduncular cistern in the direction of the prepontine cistern. The cisterns are numbered as follows: 1. Quadrigemina, 2. Interpeduncular, 3. Chiasmatica, 4. Lamina terminalis, 5. Carotid, 6. Crural (anterior ambiens), 7. Ambiens (posterior ambiens), 8. Sylvian, 9. Optocarotid sheet (optical-carotid window); 10 Anterior clinoid processes. ACA, anterior cerebral artery; AcoA, anterior communicating artery; GPe, globus pallidus externus; GPi, globus pallidus internus; ICA, internal carotid artery; MCA, middle cerebral artery; PCA, posterior cerebral artery; PcoA, posterior communicating artery. *(Continued)*

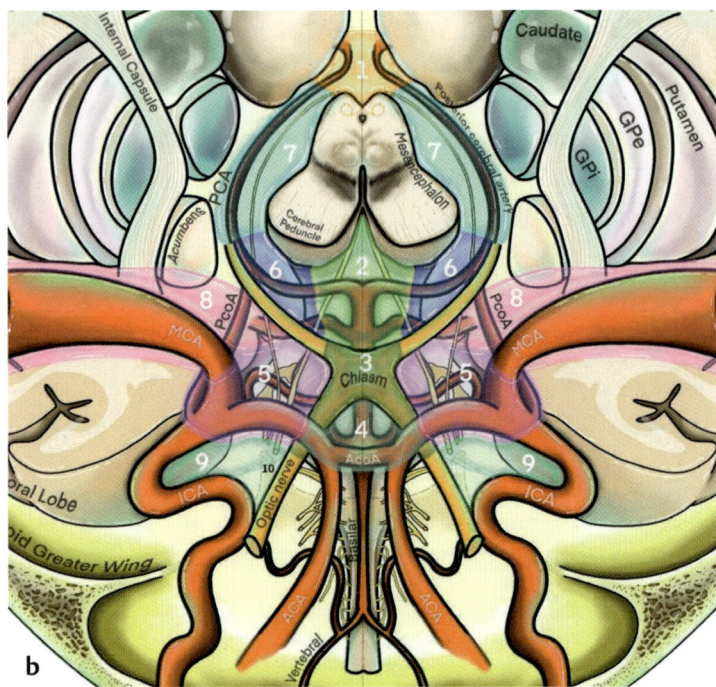

**Fig. 3.2** *(Continued)* **(b)** Overview close up to the basal cisterns. 1. Quadrigemina, 2. Interpeduncular, 3. Chiasmatica, 4. Lamina terminalis, 5. Carotid, 6. Crural (anterior ambiens), 7. Ambiens (posterior ambiens), 8. Sylvian, 9. Optocarotid sheet (optical-carotid window); 10 Anterior clinoid processes. Used with permission from Dr. Carlos Salvador Ovalle Torres.

## Anatomical Description of the Basal Cisterns

To make an easy and complete analysis, basal cisterns can be separated into "supratentorial and infratentorial" cisterns and assign a number to each of them. Cisterns can also be classified into "deep and superficial," or "paired/lateral and unpaired/midline"[8,14] cisterns to facilitate the location in determinate cases.

For academical and surgical purposes, it is also convenient to make a brief conceptual analysis of the Sylvian cistern (**Fig. 3.3**) before going further into contents. It deserves a special consideration because of many reasons:

- Its superficiality makes it an early and essential surgical landmark after opening the dura ("landmark" is defined as a remarkable anatomical structure that provides a reference for understanding the surrounding anatomy).
- It extends in the axial, coronal, and sagittal planes, with its inherited particular complexity.
- Its anatomical relationship with the basal cisterns (especially with the carotid cistern) becomes a cornerstone to gain deeper surgical elements.

## Sylvian Fissure (Lateral Sulcus) and Sylvian Cistern (Used with permission from Surgical Neurology International)[4]

The most remarkable and constant landmark in the lateral surface is the lateral sulcus (Sylvian fissure). This fissure has a superficial part and a deep part (the latter is only visible after surgical opening). As mentioned before, this is not considered as a proper basal cistern but given its extension from the lateral aspect of the brain to the medial aspect, it could be a pathway to follow in some specific cases for cisternostomy, and it has important landmarks, so its anatomy is briefly described below.

**Superficial portion:** It has a linear shape and extends from the anterior clinoid process, following the junction of the frontal with the temporal lobes. (Before the dura is opened, this same point is marked by a dense tract named orbitomeningeal band, which hides the anterior clinoid process and must be dissected to enter the subfrontal–extradural pathway.) After the dura is opened, the superficial Sylvian cistern continues without stop up to the supramarginalis gyrus. Broadly, it presents three extensions:

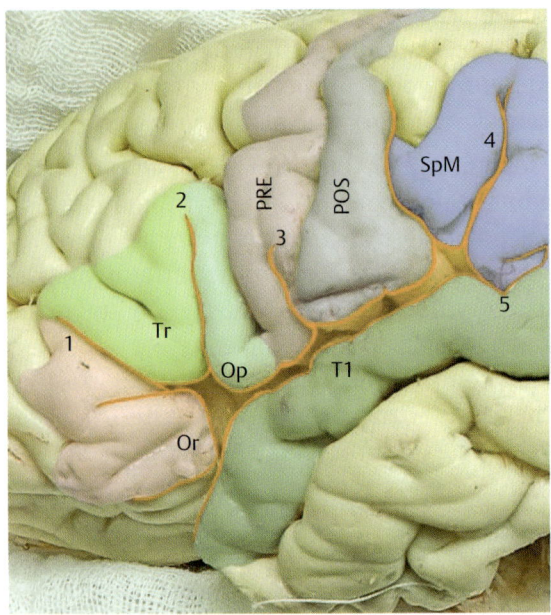

**Fig. 3.3** Sylvian fissure[15] (SF). On its lateral surface it is divided into anterior portion (A) and posterior (P) at the level of the inferior Rolandic point (intersection of the projection of the central sulcus with the SF) The lateral aspect of SF is divided in anterior ans posterior at the level of its intersection withe the central sulcus. Branches of the SF: 1: Horizontal anterior branch; 2: Anterior ascending branch; P: Posterior branch (bifurcates into terminal branches inconsistently at the level of the supramarginal gyrus); 3: Anterior subcentral sulcus (arises from the posterior ramus); Posterior subcentral groove (arises from the posterior ramus; in this specimen it is continuous with the postcentral groove); 4: Terminal ascending branch; 5: Terminal descending branch. Gyrus that delimits the FS on the lateral surface: F3: Inferior frontal gyrus (F3) subdivided into pars opercularis (Op), pars triangularis (Tr) (Landmark 1), and pars orbitalis (Or). POS, postcentral gyrus; PRE, precentral gyrus; SpM, supramarginal gyrus (surrounds proximal portion of FS and continues with T1); T1, superior temporal gyrus. Used with permission from Dr. Julio Cesar Pérez Cruz.

anterior-horizontal, anterior-vertical, and posterior. The former two confine a particular triangle-shaped portion of the inferior frontal gyrus, the pars triangularis **(Fig. 3.3)**, which is the first surgical landmark (Landmark 1). Once identified, it becomes the opening point to reach deeper levels. The arachnoid tissue bridging frontal and temporal lips separates one from the other widely at this point.[9]

**Deep portion**: It has a complex volumetrical presentation divided into two segments: the sphenoidal segment (located medially and deeper at the anterior cranial base) and the operculo-insular segment (located laterally and more superficially, directly under the superficial part of the Sylvian fissure and only visible after the surgical separation of frontal lip and temporal lip). Sphenoidal and operculo-insular segments can be divided by the presence of a particular landmark, a dense tract of white matter: the limen insulae.

**Contents:** Middle cerebral artery (MCA), lenticuloestriate arteries, polar temporal artery, superficial Sylvian vein, and deep Sylvian vein.

- Middle cerebral artery: M4 arterial branches can be followed up to M1 segment; M4 are cortical vessels at the surface up to the Sylvian frontotemporal lips; M3 from here to the circularis gyrus insulae; M2 from here up to the limen insulae (Landmark 2). At this point, there are two M1 segments (post-bifurcation, medial to the limen insulae). These two arteries come from a single trunk: the M1 pre-bifurcation segment.
- Lenticuloestriate arteries: Perforating branches mostly for the anterior perforated substance, named as early branches when from M1 pre-bifurcation.
- Polar temporal artery (temporopolar artery): Perforating branch to the temporal pole (A2 branch, after the orbitofrontal artery and the long striate artery or Heubner's recurrent artery).

- Superficial Sylvian vein: Receiving cortical veins, taking the Sylvian trajectory and finally draining to venous sinus at the sphenoid ridge (sphenopetrosal sinus).
- Deep Sylvian vein: Receives deep insular veins and drains into the sphenopetrosal sinus or directly into the cavernous sinus.

**Relationships:** At the cerebral surface, lateral sulcus (Sylvian fissure) represents the intimate contact of the inferior frontal gyrus (superior lip) and the superior temporal gyrus (inferior lip). After gentle dissection and retraction of the arachnoid bridging the two lips, lobus insularis appears. Deeper in the Sylvian valley, the limen insulae marks the start of the sphenoideal segment of the deep Sylvian fissure. The anterior perforated substance and the medial part of the pars orbitalis conform the roof in an anatomic position (in a surgical position it rests anteriorly). The floor is the planum polare. The posterior wall corresponds to a part of the uncus hippocampus. The medial wall correlates to the internal carotid artery (supraclinoid segment and its surrounding arachnoidal membrane, limit to the carotid cistern), optic tract, optic chiasma, and optic nerve. The anterior wall is incompletely marked by a thickening of the arachnoid layer just over the anterior and medial olfactory stria. At this point, the Sylvian fissure also connects with the olfactory cistern.

Once the bifurcation of M1 is noticed, the medial boundary of the deep lateral sulcus (Sylvian fissure) is almost achieved. About 8 to 15 mm further, over the M1 trajectory, an arachnoid membrane steps just in front of the supraclinoid carotid segment[4] **(Fig. 3.4).**

## The Basal Cisterns' Anatomy

It is not an easy task to describe a space and its boundaries when its walls fall down while you are describing it. This is the case of the arachnoid space: one should dissect it to describe it, and dissection eliminates the layers that outline these spaces.

In order to add new data on the anatomy of the cisterns, a detailed microscopic anatomical review was performed, making terms and concepts compatible with IFA/FIPAT. Once all cisterns were reviewed, dissection of each named arachnoid space was performed in a microanatomy laboratory. For this purpose, a specific technique was developed to visualize the arachnoid ("Rachel fluorescence technique"), which shows the dissected borders of the arachnoid tissue after cistern opening.[4]

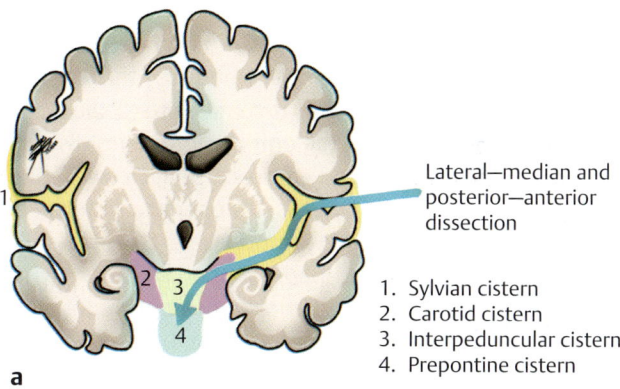

Lateral—median and posterior—anterior dissection

1. Sylvian cistern
2. Carotid cistern
3. Interpeduncular cistern
4. Prepontine cistern

a

**Fig. 3.4** Scheme of the sylvian cistern in coronal view including its components, division, and vascular content. According to Yasargil, it can be divided into four types depending on the size and the thickness of the arachnoid membrane, which determine the difficulty of surgical dissection (type 1: large, with transparent and fragile membrane; type 2: small with transparent membrane and fragile; type 3: wide with thick and resistant membrane; and type 4: small with resistant and thick membrane.[27]) **(a)** The relationship and path of the arachnoid dissection from the sylvian cistern to the interpeduncular and prepontine cisterna. *(Continued)*

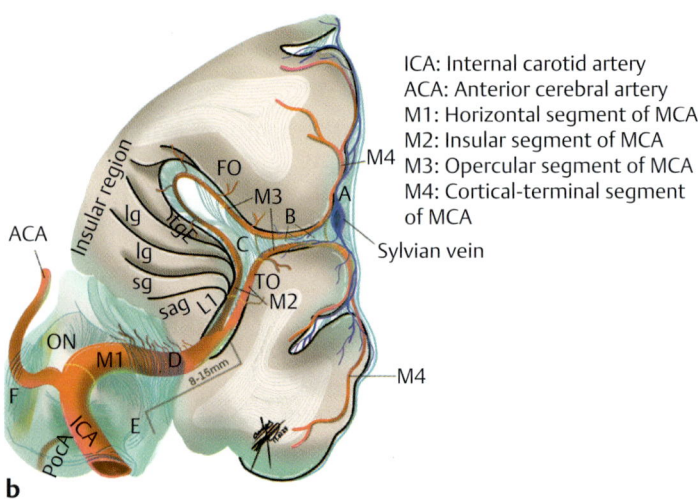

ICA: Internal carotid artery
ACA: Anterior cerebral artery
M1: Horizontal segment of MCA
M2: Insular segment of MCA
M3: Opercular segment of MCA
M4: Cortical-terminal segment
of MCA

**Fig. 3.4** *(Continued)* **(b)** the sylvian cistern is divided as follows: (A) superficial arachnoid portion, formed by the superficial arachnoid membrane, forms the external lateral wall of the sylvian cistern and demarcates the entry point during dissection, and contains the sylvian vein and cortical arteries, corresponding to the sylvian fissure and its branches; (B) opercular-intermediate portion, formed by the frontal and temporal opercula in its anterior portion and by the frontal and parietal operculi in its posterior portion, corresponding to the inferior and medial continuation of the gyri that delimit the lateral face of the sylvian fissure (specified in Fig. 3.3); adding the lateral part of the transverse gyrus of Heschl,[28] contains the M3 segment of the middle cerebral artery (MCA); (C) deepinsular portion; formed by the insula which in turn forms the medial/internal wall of the cistern with the short anterior gyrus (sag), and the short (sg) and long gyrus (lg), and the transverse gyrus of Eberstaller (tgE), contains the segment M2 and M1 post bifurcation; (D) Medial-sphenoidal portion contains the M1 segment and the lenticulostriate arteries. Used with permission from Dr. Carlos Salvador Ovalle Torres.

By joining all the pieces together (literature review, new dissections with a dedicated technique, and institutional expert-level experience at Karad University, KVV) the anatomy for a cisternostomy has been fully depicted.

In this chapter we have decided to use specific numbers for the basal cisterns in order to facilitate its study and understanding. The numbers for each of the cisterns are addressed in **Table 3.3.**

**Table 3.3** Division of the cisterns according to their tentorial relationships

| Cistern number | Cistern name | Location | Group |
|---|---|---|---|
| 1 | **Carotid** | Supratentorial/ Lateral and paired | A |
| 2 | **Chiasmatic** | Supratentorial/Midline and unpaired | |
| 3 | **Lamina terminalis** | Supratentorial/Midline and unpaired | |
| 4 | **Interpeduncular*** | Tentorial/Midline and unpaired | B |
| 5 | **Crural*** | Tentorial/Midline and unpaired | |
| 6 | **Ambiens*** | Tentorial/Lateral and paired | |
| 7 | **Quadrigeminal** | Tentorial/Midline and unpaired | |
| 8 | **Prepontine** | Infratentorial/Midline and unpaired | C |

Note: *The term "perimesencephalic cistern" is widely used. It refers to a group of cerebral cisterns around the midbrain, consisting mainly of the interpeduncular, crural, and ambiens cisterns. They are all located at the tentorial level (halfway between the supra- and infratentorial levels). This millimetric and imaginary limit could lead to some diversity in naming and defining their boundaries. In this chapter, in order to avoid unnecessary discussion, the perimesencephalic space is arbitrarily defined as "tentorial."

The authors highlight that relevant cisterns for cisternostomy procedure are: carotid, chiasmatic, lamina terminalis, interpeduncular, crural, ambiens, and prepontine.

As can be seen above, aiming to facilitate the study and understanding of the cisterns, we divide our total (eight cisterns) into three groups (A, B, and C):

- Group A is called *"the purely supratentorial cisterns"* from number 1 to 3 (carotid, chiasmatic, and lamina terminalis cisterns), which represents the pathway from the lateral aspect to the medial aspect.
- Group B is called *"the perimesencephalic cisterns"* from number 4 to 7, consisting of the central-midline pathway, from which a caudal direction should be taken.
- Group C is called *"the purely infratentorial cisterns,"* consisting of the prepontine cistern (number 8 of our list); this last cistern being the main target of the cisternostomy procedure.

## Group A: Purely Supratentorial

*The entrance to the arachnoid space*

### Carotid Cistern

The carotid cistern is formed by two sheets of arachnoid (lateral and medial), and it is contiguous medially to the lateral cerebral fossa (Sylvian cistern). It consists of a rhomboidal space surrounding the supraclinoid internal carotid artery (ICA).

The ICA should be observed underneath a thin arachnoid layer (lateral carotid sheet) (Landmark 3), just proximal to the terminal bifurcation.

- **Lateral carotid sheet:** Starting at the lateral carotid face, it goes forward (reaching the optic nerve–chiasm junction) and downward up to the IIIrd cranial nerve (oculomotor nerve). This point is important to understand the basal cistern membranes arrangement. It is named IIIrd cranial nerve cuff.[9] This arachnoid structure represents the confluence of various membranes. It must be remembered that some described membranes may not be present in part or at all because these membranes tend to be variable from one individual to another.[6,10,16]

- **Medial carotid sheet:** This layer begins once the lateral layer reaches the optic nerve. Here, with no disruption, it starts a backward pathway along the optic tract and all way down to the IIIrd cranial nerve. Thus, this membrane covers the ICA and the space between the ICA and the optic nerve (space known as the opto-carotid triangle [Landmark 4]) and covers the proximal posterior communicating artery (PcomA). This triangle serves as a window for the entrance to midline cisterns, particularly to the interpeduncular cistern[9,17] **(Fig. 3.5).**

**Contents:** ICA, posterior communicating artery (PcomA), anterior choroidal artery, and ophthalmic artery.

- Internal carotid artery: In its supraclinoid segment (intradural segment), it follows an anteromedial to posterolateral trajectory, starting at the distal dural ring.[18,19]
- Posterior communicating artery: Emerges from the posterolateral face of the ICA just next to the IIIrd cranial nerve.
- Anterior choroidal artery: Emerges from the terminal segment of the ICA, before it bifurcates into anterior and middle cerebral arteries.
- Ophthalmic artery: It has a short intradural trajectory, then it continues to the extradural space, accompanying the optic nerve into the orbit, near the emergence of the ICA from distal dural ring, beneath the medial carotid sheet.

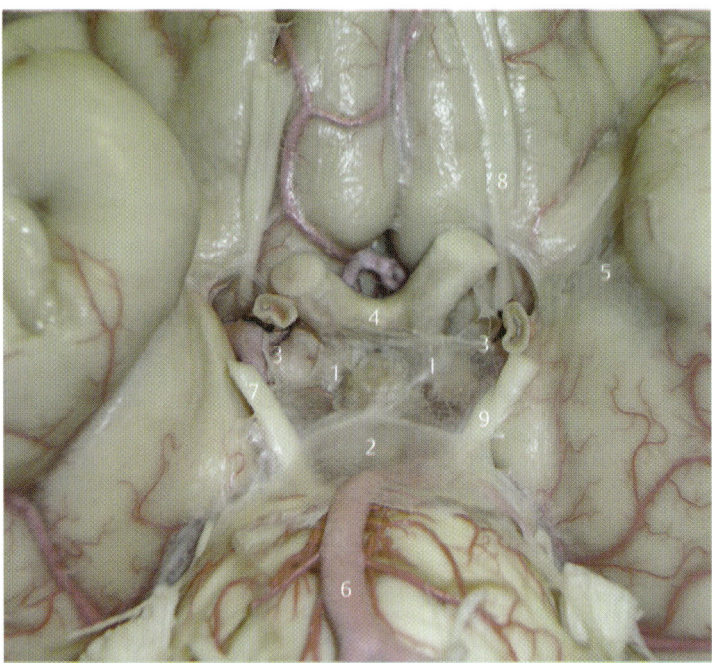

**Fig. 3.5** Basal aspect of the brain. You can see the arachnoid membranes that divide the basal cisterns as well as the main and cisternal arteries of the cranial nerves. 1. Diencephalic membrane of Liliequist, 2. Mesencephalic membrane of Liliequist (between both membranes they form the roof and floor of the interpeduncular cistern, respectively); 3. Carotid cisterna and medial carotid sheet; 4. Chiasma; 5. Sylvian fissure; 6. Basilar artery and prepontine space; 7. Oculomotor nerve; 8. Olfactory cistern; 9. IIIrd cranial nerve cistern. Used with permission from Dr. Julio Cesar Pérez Cruz.

**Relationships:** It is described rhomboid shaped. The posterior angle is represented by the IIIrd nerve cuff. The IIIrd nerve then runs in a separated cover until it continues to the lateral wall of the cavernous sinus. The anterior angle is at the optic nerve–chiasm junction, where medial and lateral sheets join. Both lateral-sided segments of the rhomboid represent the shared limit with the sphenoidal deep part of the lateral cerebral fossa (Sylvian cistern). Medial-sided segments of the rhomboid are contoured by the optic nerve, chiasm, and optic tract. They connect the carotid cistern with the cistern of the lamina terminalis (superiorly), the interpeduncular cistern (posteriorly), and the chiasmatic cistern (medially).[9,17]

## Chiasmatic Cistern

Located in the midline, the chiasmatic cistern represents a crossroads for cisternal anatomy. It connects superiorly with the cistern of the lamina terminalis, laterally with both carotid cisterns (separated by its medial sheet), and posteriorly the chiasmatic cistern is separated from the interpeduncular cistern by the Liliequist membrane.[14]

**Contents:** Optic nerves and chiasm, hypophyseal and infundibular arteries, pituitary stalk, venous plexus from optic chiasm and pituitary stalk.

**Relationships:** The optic chiasm is the main anatomic element. This structure has an anterior–superior border which represents the site of insertion for the lamina terminalis (LT). Starting here, the LT runs up and posteriorly directly to the anterior white commissure, building the posterior wall of the cistern of the LT and the anterior wall of the third ventricle. Just posterior to the optic chiasm the pituitary stalk appears, coming from diencephalic structures and going to the sellar region (pia mater and arachnoid tissue build a cylinder-shaped passage through the chiasmatic cistern, with a prior space named infundibular recess). Posterior to the pituitary stalk, a thin portion of gray matter constitutes the tuber cinereum, which is the roof of the chiasmatic cistern and part of the floor of the third ventricle (anterior to the mamillary bodies and posterior to the infundibular recess). The posterior–superior corners of the chiasmatic cistern are related directly with the PcomA and the IIIrd cranial nerve as they enter the interpeduncular cistern after they go through the carotid cistern. The posterior wall is represented by the diencephalic membrane of Liliequist.

## Lamina Terminalis Cistern

The LT membrane extends from the lower border of the anterior white commissure downward to the optic chiasm.[16,20] This membrane also has two expansions:

- **Lateral lamina terminalis membrane expansion:** From the optic chiasm to the gyrus rectus posterior part. It also has an ascending direction, making contact with the olfactory cistern.
- **Medial lamina terminalis membrane expansion:** Departing from the medial part of the gyrus rectus, it goes directly to the space between both the mesial frontal lobes. It also has a brief anterior direction with no complete fixation in its posterior part. This space is used by the anterior circulation arteries complex to pass through.

**Contents:** Optic nerves and chiasm; anterior cerebral artery A1 segment (perforating the lateral expansion membrane) and A2 segment (going through the incomplete posterior border of the medial expansion); the long striate artery (recurrent artery of Heubner) which is frequently an A1 branch; anterior communicating artery (AComA); frontopolar and superior hypophyseal branches.

**Relationships:** The cistern of the LT is located as the entrance to the peri-callosal cistern (separated from the latter by the cisternal roof, the medial expansion of LT membrane). At both sides it is separated from the carotid cistern by the lateral expansion of the LT membrane (this membrane is perforated by the A1 segment). The floor of this cistern is represented by the lower part of the LT membrane itself and the upper surface of the optic chiasm.

## Group B: The Perimesencephalic Cisterns

*The pathway of the central–midline region to the posterior–caudal direction*

### Interpeduncular Cistern

The interpeduncular cistern can be found when we visualize the ICA and identify its branch PcomA; following the PcomA (Landmark 5) in its medial aspect, it must be dissected and trespassed to reach this midline cistern, passing above the IIIrd nerve and going in perpendicular direction to the Liliequist membrane.

It is well known that perimesencephalic structures correspond to the tentorial notch (tentorial incisura) level. This space is the theoretical limit and real pathway of communication between supra- and infratentorial spaces. Thus, reaching this cistern not only serves as an access to the midline but also to find a connection to infratentorial levels.

The tentorial notch (incisura) is classically divided into an anterior, middle, and posterior parts.[9,10,21] Each one has a particular cistern associated: interpeduncular cistern (anterior part), cistern ambiens (middle part), and quadrigeminal cistern (posterior part) **(Fig. 3.6a, b)**. The anterior part has an important element, which constitutes both upper and lower limits of the interpeduncular cistern: the Liliequist membrane.

The Liliequist membrane may be understood as a projection formed by an arachnoid membrane extending from the dorsum sellae to the mammillary bodies.[22] It covers the dorsum sellae; this arachnoid layer then extends laterally to both posterior clinoidal processes, and finally

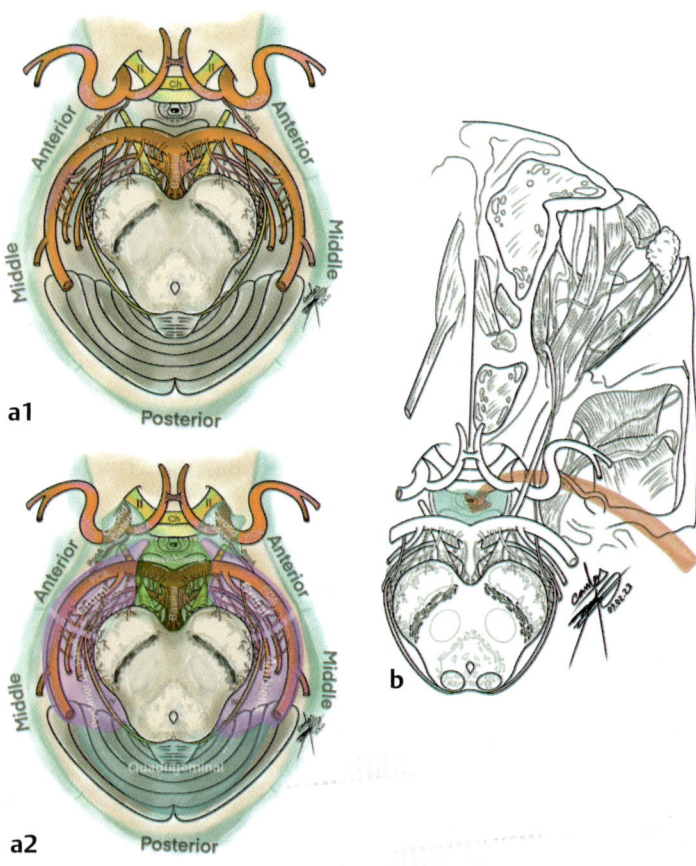

**Fig. 3.6 (a)** Segmentation of the tentorial notch and its relationship of the division with the perimesencephalic cisterns (blue purple and green shaded) and the carotid cistern (light blue shaded). ACA, anterior cerebral artery; AcoA, anterior communicating artery; Ch, chiasm; MCA, middle cerebral artery; PCA, posterior cerebral artery; PcoA, posterior communicating artery; II, III, and IV cranial nerves. **(b)** Expanded and simplified view diagram showing the anatomical route to follow (red arrow) to reach the interpeduncular cistern (light blue shading) following the path of the greater wing of the sphenoid, and then through the carotid optic window. Used with permission from Dr. Carlos Salvador Ovalle Torres.

runs posteriorly in the search of the brainstem. As soon as this membrane leaves the posterior clinoidal process (with its posteriorly oriented trajectory), it spreads into two membranes[4] **(Fig. 3.7):**

- **Diencephalic membrane:** Continuing in a slightly posterior–superior direction (with intimate adhesion to the IIIrd nerve cuff at both sides), this membrane finally arrives at brainstem levels. Here, it attaches to mamillary bodies. This membrane is thick, regular, and uniform along its surface, forming the roof of the interpeduncular cistern. When this membrane is surgically perforated (i.e., while making an endoscopic ventriculocisternostomy of the third ventricle, after

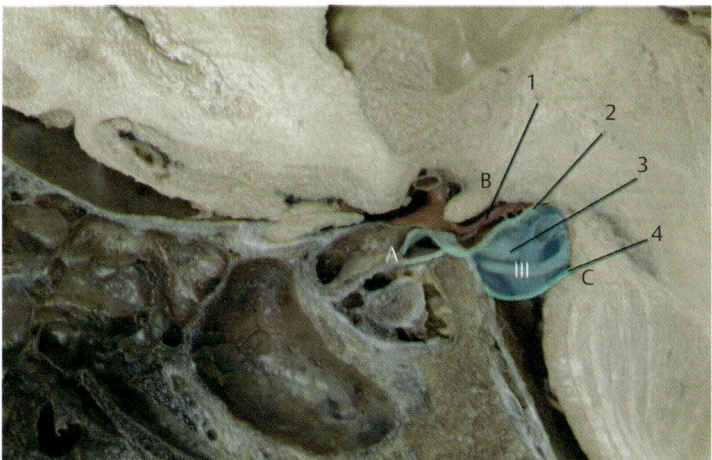

**Fig. 3.7** Insertion of Liliequist membrane, parallel to the posterior communicating artery (1) from the dorsum of the sella (A); toward the base of the mammillary bodies (B) the diencephalic membrane (2) is inserted, and toward the pontomesencephalic sulcus (C), the mesencephalic membrane is inserted, forming the interpeduncular cistern (blue shaded), in intimate relationship with the cranial nerve III. (3) the level of the basilar tip and its bifurcation, (4) mesencephalic membrane. Used with permission from Dr. Julio Cesar Pérez Cruz.

the tuber cinereum is traversed), the third ventricle and basal cisterns are then communicated. After this perforation, basilar artery should be easily seen among arachnoid trabeculae and beneath the mesencephalic membrane.[22-24]

- **Mesencephalic membrane:** From the same anterior insertion as the diencephalic membrane, this one instead runs in an oblique manner (in a posterior–inferior direction). Once at the brainstem level, it attaches to the pontomesencephalic sulcus, just above the tip and bifurcation of the basilar artery. Posterior communicating artery (PcomA) should be encountered here, finalizing its trajectory, dividing P1 from P2 segment of the posterior cerebral artery (PCA). Laterally, the medial carotid sheet, descending up to the oculomotor nerve cuff, joins the mesencephalic membrane of Liliequist. It continues as a single membrane over the pontomesencephalic sulcus (forming the lateral pontomesencephalic membrane). The Liliequist mesencephalic membrane is very thin and mostly incomplete, but it has several attachments to the oculomotor nerve and PcomA sheath.

**Contents:** Basilar artery tip and bifurcation, posterior communicating artery (PcomA), posterior cerebral artery (PCA), superior cerebellar artery (SCA), oculomotor nerve, venous complex.

- Basilar tip and bifurcation (Landmark 6): This arterial complex is exactly situated where the mesencephalic membrane starts its insertion. Just a few millimeters downward, dissecting arachnoid space, the prepontine cistern is reached.
- Posterior communicating artery (PcomA): This artery can be seen coming from the carotid cistern (serving as a guide for dissection). It arrives and ends at the P1–P2 level of the PCA **(Fig. 3.6)**.

- Posterior cerebral artery (PCA) and superior cerebellar artery (SCA): Mesencephalic membrane insertion involves both the arteries, side to side of the midbrain anterior surface, marked laterally by the apparent origin of the oculomotor nerve. The later nerve passes inferiorly to the PCA and superiorly to the SCA, lateral to the upper portion of the basilar artery.
- Oculomotor nerve: This nerve can be seen up to its apparent origin at the middle portion of the mesencephalic peduncles surface (sulcus of the oculomotor nerve). It passes between PCA and SCA before entering to the wall of the cavernous sinus and continues anteriorly (cisternal portion) till it enters to the superior–lateral wall of the dura of the cavernous sinus.
- Venous complex: It includes drainage veins from posterior communicating, pontomesencephalic, and thalamoperforating veins.

**Relationships:** The membrane of Liliequist is a partially trabecular, partially dense, folded inner arachnoid membrane, and the most important anatomic landmark in the approach to the interpeduncular fossa, and sellar and parasellar regions.[25] The roof of this cistern is composed by the mamillary bodies and the diencephalic membrane of Liliequist. This roof is directly situated behind the chiasmatic cistern. Only a thin layer of gray matter (the tuber cinereum, part of the floor of the third ventricle; point of perforation for the previously named endoscopic ventriculocisternostomy of the third ventricle) is situated between this cistern and the third ventricle above. On both sides, the cistern ambiens occupy the middle aspect of the tentorial incisura. The posterior perforated substance (perforated by small branches of the basilar and P1 arteries) is at the back of the interpeduncular cistern. Downward, beyond the incomplete mesencephalic membrane of Liliequist, the cisternal space is continued by the prepontine cistern.

## Crural Cistern

Classical anatomic references describe this cistern as located in front of the ambiens cistern and just lateral to the interpeduncularis cistern. Nevertheless, the FIPAT/IFA nomenclature does not name it particularly. Crural cistern is a paired cistern at the tentorial/mesencephalic level, midway between interpenduncularis and ambiens ones. The anterior choroidal artery (as an anterolateral limit with the carotid cistern) and the PcomA (as posteromedial limit with the interpeduncularis cistern) demarcate the crural cistern location.[6,10,16] Crural and cistern ambiens together can be denominated as a single cistern named "lateral mesencephalic cistern" or "ambiens cistern" with its posterior portion being the ambiens cistern itself and the anterior portion corresponding to the crural cistern.[26] The crural membrane[3] (separating ambiens from crural cistern) must be differentiated from the intracrural membrane[26] (separating crural cistern in superior and inferior compartments), both appearing as incomplete, and it is important to remind that these membranes may not be constant.[6,10,13,16]

**Contents:** Anterior choroidal artery (last branch of carotid before bifurcation), posterior choroidal artery (PCA branch), P2a segment of the PCA, and proximal part of the basal vein of Rosenthal.

**Relationships:** The anterior and mid part of the uncus form its lateral boundary; the division between mid and posterior portion of the uncus is marked by an arachnoid layer running from lateral to medial: the lateral pontomesencephalic membrane (this membrane continues up to the IIIrd nerve cuff; then it runs downward as the anterior pontine membrane). This same membrane, once it gets near the VIth cranial nerve, at the ponto-medullaris junction, starts a lateral trajectory as the lateral ponto-medullaris membrane,

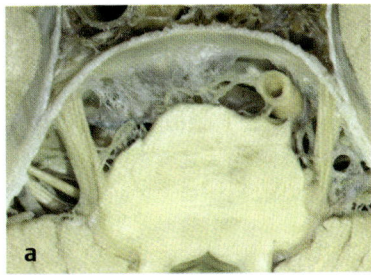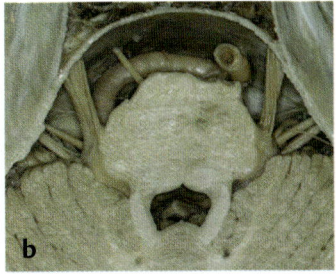

**Fig. 3.8 (a)** The pontomedullary membrane is observed corresponding to the lower limit of the prepontine cistern, part of its content corresponding to the anterior inferior cerebellar artery (AICA) and the basilar artery; the Dorello canal is observed. Laterally on both sides of the pontomedullary membrane, part of the content of the pontocerebellar cystern is observed, including the trigeminal nerves and complex of VII–VIII cranial nerves. **(b)** The pontomedullary membrane has been removed, exposing a dolicho path of the basilar artery, as well as the path of the VIth cranial nerve, as well as part of the fourth ventricle in the posterior region. Used with permission from Dr. Julio Cesar Pérez Cruz.

just up to the IXth cranial nerve; at this point this membrane blends with the exterior cerebellar arachnoid membrane (**Fig. 3.8**).

From the mentioned posterior uncus point, another thin membrane (the intracrural membrane) runs anteromedially dividing crural cistern into a superior (dorsal) and inferior (ventral) compartments, where the anterior choroidal artery and PcomA can be found, respectively; however, this membrane may be present or absent variably. The medial wall of the cistern is the lateral surface of the mesencephalon.

## Ambiens Cistern

The compartment between the mesial surface of the temporal lobe (uncus posterior part, parahippocampus, dentate gyrus, fornix and fimbria) and the lateral surface of the mesencephalon (from the lateral edge of the quadrigeminal plate) takes the name of ambiens cistern. Anteriorly, it limits with the intercrural cistern. But both crural and ambiens cisterns can be considered as a single, "ambiens cistern" being the anterior portion of the ambiens cistern equal to the crural cistern as it is mentioned above. Posteriorly, it limits with the quadrigeminal cistern. It forms part of the basal cisterns belonging to the "perimesencephalic cisterns" but in the issue that concerns now, this loses relevance because this territory is not of surgical interest during cisternostomy procedure; therefore, it is only briefly described.

**Contents:** Posterior cerebral artery (P2–P3 segments), SCA, choroidal posterior–lateral arteries, basal vein, IVth cranial nerve (trochlear nerve).

## Quadrigeminal Cistern

As mentioned above in the same way as that of the ambiens cistern, the quadrigeminal cistern is also a part of the group of "perimesencephalic" basal cisterns, located posterior to the midbrain; therefore, it is also not considered to be of surgical interest for the cisternostomy procedure, and it will also be described briefly.

It is found by following the pericallosal cistern posteriorly and caudally. The pineal gland and quadrigeminal plate are reached just behind–below the splenium of the corpus callosum.

**Contents:** Posterior cerebral artery (P3 segment), quadrigeminal arteries, choroidal posterior–medial arteries, SCA, internal cerebral vein, basal vein, vein of Galeno, IVth cranial nerve (trochlear nerve).

## The Purely Infratentorial Cisterns

*The end of the pathway "the basal cisternostomy target"*

## Prepontine Cistern

The midline/unpaired cisterns, from the tentorium down, are: interpeduncularis, prepontine, and pre-medullary cisterns.

This is the only cistern included in our last group and as its name suggests, the prepontine cistern is located anterior to the pons, and the superior portion of this cistern represents the main target territory to place the tip of a drainage catheter under the microscopic vision during the basal cisternostomy procedure, achieving the communication and drainage of CSF from the supratentorial and infratentorial cisterns.

In the section on the relationships and extension of the crural cistern, we described the membranes where the prepontine cistern is properly situated, remembering that it is between the right and left anterior pontine membranes. Superiorly, it is related to the interpeduncularis cistern and inferiorly it continues to the pre-medullary cistern.

**Contents:** The main structure located as a central axis is the trunk of the basilar artery. The VIth cranial nerve (abducens) and all its trajectory pointing to the abducens nerve canal or Dorello canal. The anterior inferior cerebellar artery (AICA) also starts here, with some perforating pontine arteries and pontine veins (**Fig. 3.8a, b**).

**Relationships:** The anterior surface of this cistern is related to the clivus; posteriorly it is related to the pons and its centrally located element, the basilar artery in its trajectory over the basilar sulcus. The mesencephalic membrane of Liliequist represents the roof. At the floor of this cistern, a thickened membrane (where the vertebral arteries join to originate the basilar artery, approximately at the ponto-medullaris junction) separates the prepontine cistern from the premedullaris cistern. Finally, bilateral to the prepontine cistern we find the cerebellopontine cisterns with their respective neurovascular content.

## Discussion

For the neurosurgeon, knowledge of the basal cisterns is essential to ensure reaching the goal of neurological preservation while getting deeper into the brain (**Fig. 3.9a, b**).

The cisternal corridors are not only the routes but also containers for arteries, veins, and nerves, needing dissection of the arachnoid membranes, allowing opening of cisterns and drainage of CSF causing an immediate "relaxation" effect. This procedure has been practiced routinely in brain aneurysm surgeries and brain tumor resections. The same concept is now applied to cisternal opening and CSF drainage for severe brain trauma.

Talking about the cisternostomy procedure itself, pterional and frontotemporal approaches allow to gain access to the previously mentioned anatomy, not only to show the corresponding elements, but also to diminish as much of parenchymal manipulation as possible and appropriate vision angles. Therefore, anatomical knowledge of this complex cisternal system facilitates performing the external basal cisternostomy procedure, managing cerebral edema based on anatomical and physiological basis.

Thorough knowledge of the microscopic anatomy is a sine-qua-non for a proper and safe cisternal managing. Landmarks recognition and tri-dimensional orientation are mandatory, as well as microsurgical skills. All of these topics, once understood with lectures and classes, could and should be learned/trained efficiently at the laboratory.[15] Simulation builds good operators (at a safe scenario) as much as surgical procedures builds good surgeons (at the stressful and demanding operating room).

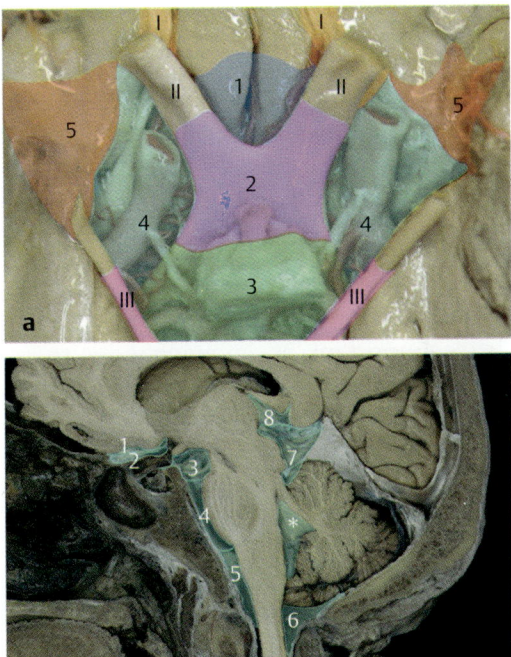

**Fig. 3.9** **(a)** Basal aspect of the brain focused on the basal cisterns, their limits, and their content. 1. Lamina terminalis cistern; 2. Chiasmatic cistern; 3. Interpeduncular cistern (in this dissection, the pituitary stalk and the pituitary gland have been preserved, so they are ventral to the chiasmatic and interpeduncular cistern, respectively, without actually forming part of its content; below the pituitary gland you can see the basilar artery and its bifurcation); 4. Carotid cistern (note that at the level of the marking number corresponding to this cistern the origin of the posterior communicating artery is evident); 5. Citerna Silviana; I, olfactory cistern; II, optic nerve; III, cistern of the IIIrd cranial nerve. **(b)** Complementary view of anatomical dissection of the midline cisterns (unpaired cisterns). 1. Lamina terminalis cisterna; 2. Chiasmatic cistern; 3. Interpeduncular cistern; 4. Prepontine cistern; 5. Premedullary cistern; 6. Magna cistern; 7. Quadrigeminal cistern; 8. Interposito veil cistern; *, Fourth ventricle. Used with permission from Dr. Julio Cesar Pérez Cruz.

## Conclusion

The first step to master a surgical technic is mastering the basis of its anatomy. In this particular case of cisternostomy, the anatomical facts confronted by the surgeon are detailed and complex. This anatomical review is cornerstone to perform it safely and effectively, because surgical results and anatomic–physiological basis are deeply related.

The final localization of the tip of a core-cistern-drainage catheter is as important as knowing how to reach this particular arachnoid space, how to precisely determine this position, and how to navigate between their elements, which does not allow for any mistakes.

## References

1. Cherian I, Yi G, Munakomi S. Cisternostomy: replacing the age old decompressive hemicraniectomy? Asian J Neurosurg 2013;8(3):132–138
2. Elsawaf Y, Anetsberger S, Luzzi S, Elbabaa SK. Early decompressive craniectomy as management for severe traumatic brain injury in the pediatric population: a comprehensive literature review. World Neurosurg 2020;138:9–18
3. Cherian I, Grasso G, Bernardo A, Munakomi S. Anatomy and physiology of cisternostomy. Chin J Traumatol 2016;19(1):7–10
4. Villanueva P, Baldoncini M, Forlizzi V, et al. Microneurosurgical anatomy of the basal cisterns: a brief review for cisternostomy. Surg Neurol Int 2023;14:97
5. Ettmüller ME, Ruysch F. Epistola Anatomica, Problematica duodecima, Authore Mich. Ernesto Ettmullero, M. D. &c. Ad Virum Clarissimum Fredericum Ruyschium Med. Doct. Anatomiae ac Botanices Professorem. De Cerebri Corticali substantia, &c. Karnataka: Clear Prints; 1699
6. Yasargil MG, Kasdaglis K, Jain KK, Weber HP. Anatomical observations of the subarachnoid cisterns of the brain during surgery. J Neurosurg 1976;44(3):298–302

7. Federative International Programme for Anatomical Terminology. Terminology. Terminologia Anatomica. 2nd ed. Rio de Janeiro: Federative International Programme for Anatomical Terminology; 2019

8. Altafulla J, Bordes S, Jenkins S, et al. The basal subarachnoid cisterns: surgical and anatomical considerations. World Neurosurg 2019;129:190–199

9. Rhoton AL. Surgeons CoN. Rhoton's Cranial Anatomy and Surgical Approaches: Oxford: Oxford University Press; 2019

10. Yasargil MG. Microneurosurgery. Microsurgical Anatomy of the Basal Cisterns and Vessels of the Brain, Diagnostic Studies, General Operative Techniques and Pathological Considerations of the Intracranial Aneurysms. Vol. 1. United States: Thieme; 1984

11. Alperin N, Bagci AM, Lee SH, Lam BL. Automated quantitation of spinal CSF volume and measurement of craniospinal CSF redistribution following lumbar withdrawal in idiopathic intracranial hypertension. AJNR Am J Neuroradiol 2016;37(10): 1957–1963

12. Sakka L, Coll G, Chazal J. Anatomy and physiology of cerebrospinal fluid. Eur Ann Otorhinolaryngol Head Neck Dis 2011;128(6):309–316

13. Lü J, Zhu XL. Characteristics of distribution and configuration of intracranial arachnoid membranes. Surg Radiol Anat 2005;27(6):472–481

14. Rai S, Srivastava S, Kamath M, Murlimanju BV, Parmar G, Chebrolu G. Delineation of subarachnoid cisterns using CT cisternography, CT brain positive and negative contrast, and a three dimensional MRI sequence: a pictorial review. Cureus 2022;14(4):e23741

15. Ovalle Torres CS, Espinosa Mora A, Campero A, Cherian I, Sufianov A, Fragoza Sanchez E, et al. Enhancing microsurgical skills in neurosurgery residents of low-income countries: A comprehensive guide. Surg Neurol Int. 2023;14:437

16. Inoue K, Seker A, Osawa S, Alencastro LF, Matsushima T, Rhoton AL Jr. Microsurgical and endoscopic anatomy of the supratentorial arachnoidal membranes and cisterns. Neurosurgery 2009;65(4):644–664, discussion 665

17. Adib SD, Herlan S, Ebner FH, Hirt B, Tatagiba M, Honegger J. Interoptic, trans-lamina terminalis, opticocarotid triangle, and caroticosylvian windows from mini-supraorbital, frontomedial, and pterional perspectives: a comparative cadaver study with artificial lesions. Front Surg 2019;6:40

18. Bouthillier A, van Loveren HR, Keller JT. Segments of the internal carotid artery: a new classification. Neurosurgery 1996;38(3):425–432, discussion 432–433

19. Gibo H, Lenkey C, Rhoton AL Jr. Microsurgical anatomy of the supraclinoid portion of the internal carotid artery. J Neurosurg 1981;55(4):560–574

20. Tubbs RS, Nguyen HS, Loukas M, Cohen-Gadol AA. Anatomic study of the lamina terminalis: neurosurgical relevance in approaching lesions within and around the third ventricle. Childs Nerv Syst 2012;28(8):1149–1156

21. Testut L, Latarjet A, Latarjet M, Devy G, Dupret S. Tratado de Anatomia Humana: Salvat Editores, S.A.; 1949

22. Dias DA, Castro FL, Yared JH, Lucas Júnior A, Ferreira Filho LA, Ferreira NF. Liliequist membrane: radiological evaluation, clinical and therapeutic implications. Radiol Bras 2014;47(3):182–185

23. Abdalá-Vargas NJ, Cifuentes-Lobelo HA, Ordoñez-Rubiano E, et al. Anatomic variations of the floor of the third ventricle: surgical implications for endoscopic third ventriculostomy. Surg Neurol Int 2022;13:218

24. Dezena RA. Surgical Technique of Endoscopic Third Ventriculostomy (ETV). Endoscopic Third Ventriculostomy: Classic Concepts and a State-of-the-Art Guide. Cham: Springer International Publishing; 2020:81–91

25. Lü J, Zhu X. Microsurgical anatomy of the interpeduncular cistern and related arachnoid membranes. J Neurosurg 2005;103(2):337–341

26. Jessen NA, Munk AS, Lundgaard I, Nedergaard M. The glymphatic system: a beginner's guide. Neurochem Res 2015;40(12):2583–2599

27. García Navarro V, Castillo Velázquez GA. Opening of the Silvian valley. In Strategies and approaches in cranial neurosurgery. Vol.I. Amolca Publishing House; 2015:211

28. Campero Á, Ajler P. Cerebral sulci and gyri. In Surgical neuroanatomy. Vol. I. Journal Editions. 2019:6

# The Physiology and Understanding of Cisternostomy

**4**

*Hira Burhan and Iype Cherian*

## Anatomy of Cisternostomy

Cisternostomy is a micro-neurosurgical procedure requiring the understanding of the skull base anatomy and the intricate skills needed for fine microsurgical procedures. The suprasellar cistern, also referred to as the chiasmatic cistern or pentagon of basal cisterns, is a fluid-filled space containing cerebrospinal fluid (CSF). It is situated above the sella turcica, beneath the hypothalamus, and between the temporal lobe unci. Within this cistern are the proximal segment of the Sylvian fissure, the optic chiasm, the infundibular stalk, and the circle of Willis, which consists of interconnected cerebrovascular arteries. It is continuous posteriorly with the interpeduncular cistern. Reaching the suprasellar cistern in such an intricate anatomical location is a challenge in a tight, aggressive brain. Approaching the cistern through the base of the skull and opening it to the atmospheric pressure is the anatomical basis of cisternostomy.[1]

# "Brain Unlocking"—the Anatomical Concept

The concept of brain "unlocking" is pivotal in microsurgical procedures. The brain resembles a tube that folds across three dimensions: sagittal, axial, and oblique planes. Employing a pterional approach with sylvian dissection partially unfolds the brain obliquely. However, this maneuver restricts the surgeon to a single surgical perspective (**Fig. 4.1**). Maneuvers to unlock the brain in the sagittal and axial planes gives an excellent exposure to the skull base.

The dura of the frontal and the temporal lobes is adherent to each other, and the anterior clinoid process can be "buried and hidden" between these two lobes. "Unlocking" of these

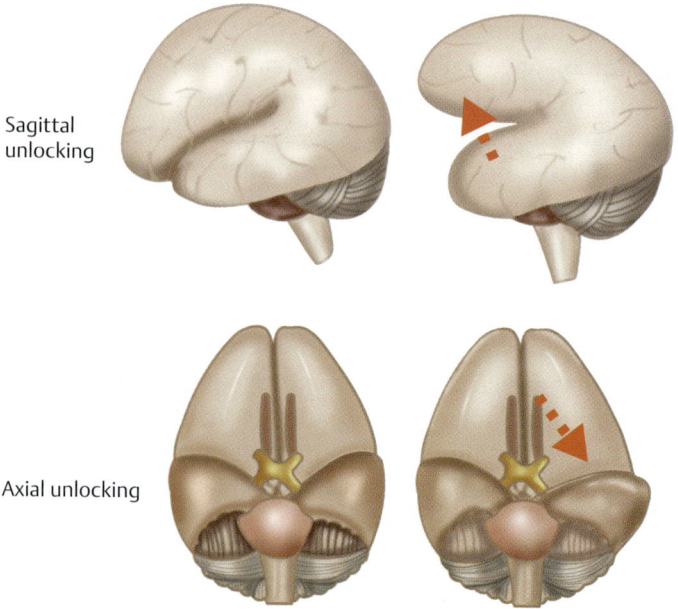

Sagittal unlocking

Axial unlocking

**Fig. 4.1** Schematic diagram of brain unlocking.

lobes is particularly important for approaching the basal cisterns, which is provided by incising the orbito-meningeal band (OMB) in the sagittal and axial planes (**Fig. 4.2a, b**).

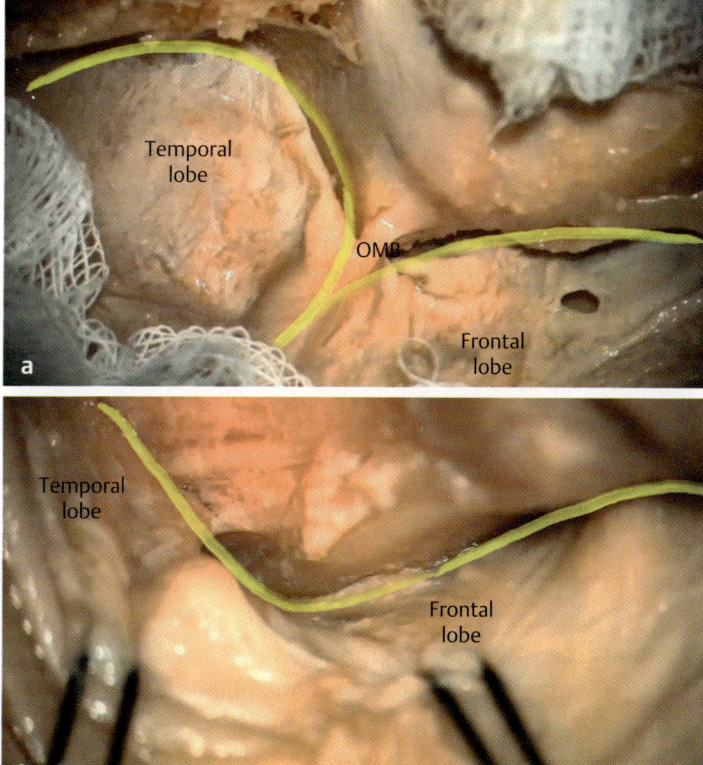

**Fig. 4.2** **(a)** Before orbito-meningeal band (OMB) dissection. Notice the adherent frontal and temporal lobe. **(b)** After OMB dissection. Notice the flattening of the tight curve. Based on Video 12.1 from Cherian I, Burhan H. Skull base approaches to the lesions of sellar and parasellar regions: anatomy, techniques, and insights. In: Janakiram N. eds. Atlas of Sellar, Suprasellar, and Parasellar Lesions. Thieme; 2022.

To achieve sagittal unlocking of the brain, extensive removal of the sphenoid ridge is necessary. For axial unlocking of the temporal lobe, the temporal lobe must be extradurally detached from the cavernous sinus, thereby opening its curve **(Fig. 4.2)**. Integrating sylvian dissection with these techniques significantly enhances basal exposure by laterally obliquely opening the brain. However, in cases of tightly packed traumatic brain injury, performing sylvian dissection may not be feasible, although axial and sagittal unlocking techniques can still be employed to access the brain's base.

Once the dura mater is exposed, extensive drilling of the sphenoid ridge and temporal bone is performed to achieve maximal separation of the frontal lobe from the temporal lobe in a sagittal direction. This maneuver allows for a significant view of the skull base. The OMB is located at the junction of the basi-frontal and temporal lobes, positioned laterally along the superior orbital fissure.

Sharp dissection of the OMB allows to view the true cavernous membrane. This membrane hosts the neuro-vascular structures of the cavernous sinuses, hence making it an important structure when dissecting in the region. Upon reaching true cavernous membrane plane, a sharp dissection can be performed in a peri-cavernous plane **(Fig. 4.3)**. At the level of V2 and below, this plane is absent, but the interdural plane may be maintained, thereby decreasing the bleeding. This approach is a modification of the traditional Dolenc,[2] as it ensures the intact true cavernous membrane (TCM) throughout the peri-cavernous dissection, preventing the bleeding that otherwise occurs in the Dolenc approach. If the bleeding occurs, fibrin glue and surgicel can be used to overcome it.[3,4] However, care must be taken with the injection volume of fibrin as it may cause change in the venous drainage pattern with subsequent venous congestion.[5]

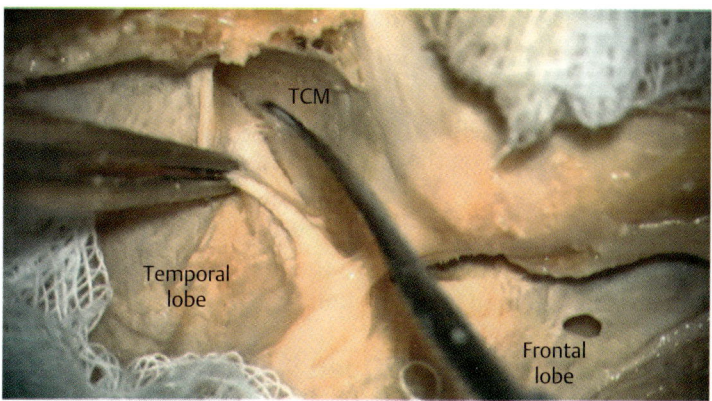

**Fig. 4.3** Orbito-meningeal band (OMB) dissection and visualization of the true cavernous membrane. TCM, true cavernous membrane. Based on Video 12.1 from Cherian I, Burhan H. Skull base approaches to the lesions of sellar and parasellar regions: anatomy, techniques, and insights. In: Janakiram N. eds. Atlas of Sellar, Suprasellar, and Parasellar Lesions. Thieme; 2022.

## A Simple Classification of the Carotid in Relation to Cisternostomy

The study of the internal carotid artery is crucial to learning skull base surgery. Providing two-thirds of the cerebral circulation, the internal carotid artery follows a tortuous course as it ascends from the bifurcation of the common carotid in the neck, into the cranium, running extradurally along the two sides of the cranial base, until it reaches the distal dural ring. From here, the internal carotid artery follows an intra-dural course. Throughout its course, the internal carotid artery takes sharp turns at almost right angles to its segments,[6] illustrating a relationship to adjacent bony and neurovascular structures of the skull base. These anatomical landmarks assist in identifying each segment and its spatial position within the skull base. Over the years, various classifications have been proposed to divide the carotid artery into segments, ranging from simpler to more complex systems based on their intended utility. These classifications are based on angiography,[2] cadaveric neuroanatomy,[3,4] and vertical endoscopic views.[7] The authors propose a very simple model based on the fact that odd segments are vertical and even segments are horizontal—minor modification of the classification proposed by Professor Fukushima.[8] This learning model is based on the author's observations in more than 50 human cadaver skull base dissections.

## The Carotid Segments—Open Skull Base

To better comprehend carotid anatomy, a simplified two-dimensional model is employed, categorizing segments based on vertical and horizontal orientations. These segments are numbered in the opposite direction of blood flow, starting distally and moving proximally. Vertical segments are assigned odd numbers, while horizontal segments are assigned even numbers. Each segment is named according to its relationship with adjacent structures, as depicted in **Figs. 4.4** and **4.5**.

Thus, the extradural internal carotid can be classified into the following segments:

- C7: Cervical segment or para-pharyngeal segment.
- C6: Petrosal segment.
- C5: Paraclival segment.
- C4: Cavernous horizontal segment.
- C3: Paraclinoid or parasellar segment.
- C2: Intradural segment.

The tortuous course by the carotid artery and its intimate extradural relationship to the skull base structures make it crucial to fully understand it. This simple method will help young neurosurgeons to identify the carotid segments with respect to horizontal and vertical planes and important

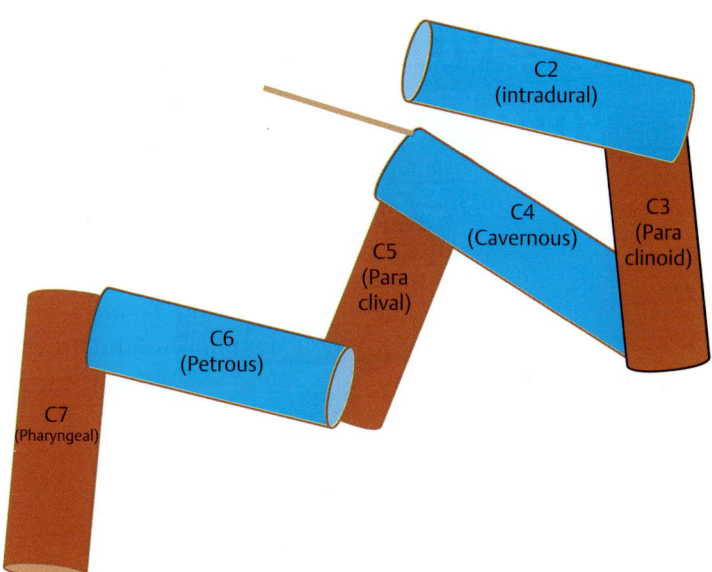

**Fig. 4.4** Nomenclature of carotid segments in relation to adjacent structures. The horizontal and vertical orientation of even and odd segments can be seen. Reproduced from Cherian I, Burhan H. Skull base approaches to the lesions of sellar and parasellar regions: anatomy, techniques, and insights. In: Janakiram N. eds. Atlas of Sellar, Suprasellar, and Parasellar Lesions. Thieme; 2022.

landmarks, which will be helpful to perform complex microsurgical procedures like cisternostomy, preventing damage to the internal carotid artery. It should, however, be noted that anatomical variants do exist between patients and care needs to be taken to identify and respect the variant anatomy for best surgical results.

## Peri-cavernous Anatomy: The Anterior and Posterior Clinoid

Once the OMB is dissected under high magnification, the flattening of cerebral gyri becomes evident. This creates

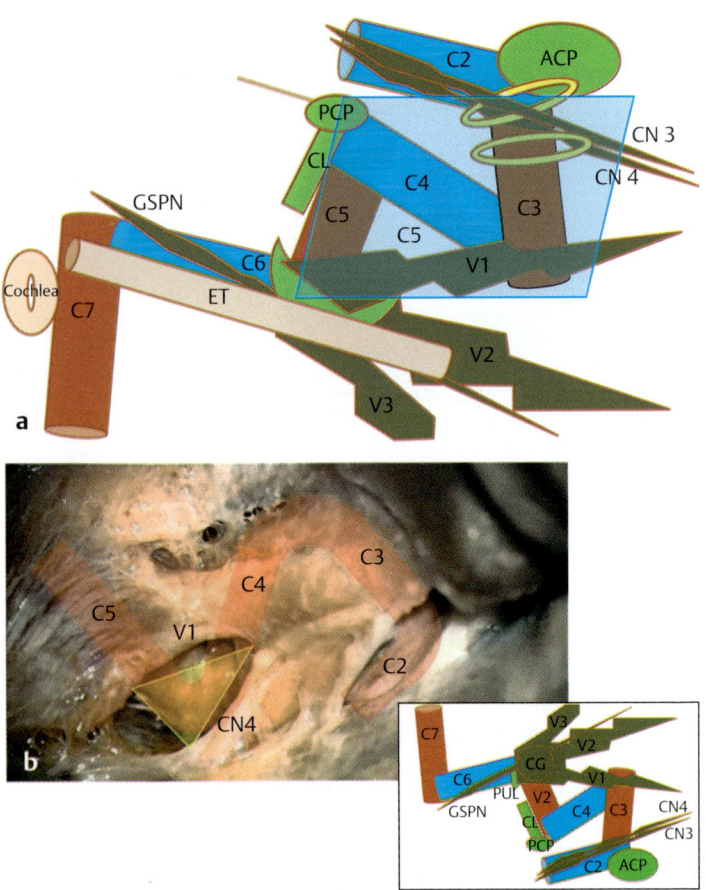

**Fig. 4.5** The extradural course of internal carotid in relation to the adjacent structures. **(a)** The illustration of the structures in a 2 dimensional plane. **(b)** Maps the illustration onto a cadaveric dissection view showing the curve of the internal carotid. Note the close relationship of the cochlea posterolateral to the carotid curve from C7 to C6. ACP: Anterior clinoid process; GSPN: Greater superior petrosal nerve; PCP: Posterior clinoid process. Reproduced from Cherian I, Burhan H. Skull base approaches to the lesions of sellar and parasellar regions: anatomy, techniques, and insights. In: Janakiram N. eds. Atlas of Sellar, Suprasellar, and Parasellar Lesions. Thieme; 2022.

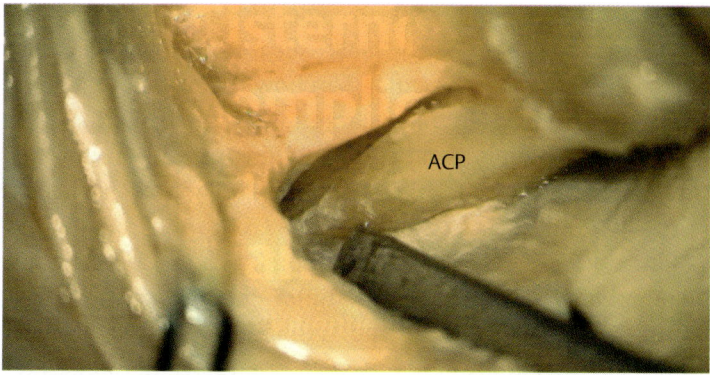

**Fig. 4.6** The ACP visualized after orbito-meningeal band (OMB) dissection. ACP: Anterior clinoid process. Based on Video 12.1 from Cherian I, Burhan H. Skull base approaches to the lesions of sellar and parasellar regions: anatomy, techniques, and insights. In: Janakiram N. eds. Atlas of Sellar, Suprasellar, and Parasellar Lesions. Thieme; 2022.

a plane where the dura covering the frontal lobe can be dissected from the anterior clinoid process, and the dura covering the temporal lobe can be separated from the true cavernous membrane of the cavernous sinus.

This maneuver exposes the anterior clinoid process, facilitating easier anterior clinoidectomy. Additionally, it allows the temporal lobe to be displaced laterally in an extradural manner, enabling axial unlocking and peri-cavernous peeling, as illustrated in **Fig. 4.6**.

# The Physiology of Cisternostomy

## The Pathophysiology of Brain Edema—the CSF Shift Edema

Like any other fluid, the CSF cannot be compressed fully. One can only wonder where this 120 mL of CSF, which resides in the basal cisterns, goes in a traumatic brain. A pathway for this CSF to "leak" out from the basal cisterns is through the paravascular Virchow Robin spaces which are seen as swollen or enlarged in radiological imaging for various brain pathologies including brain trauma. In a subarachnoid hemorrhage, the AQP4 channels lining the Virchow Robin spaces allow for the CSF to move out of the subarachnoid cisterns to accommodate the blood from the hemorrhage. The CSF then "shifts" into the paravascular brain spaces, increasing the axonal spaces, resulting in brain edema. Experiments in mice brain have demonstrated this pathogenesis which initiates a sequence of events in brain edema.

## Reversing the CSF Shift—Cisternal Drainage

Brain edema, followed by decompression with bone flap removal, aggravates the damage done to the cerebral tissue. The inter-axonal space, now occupied by the leaked CSF from basal cisterns, distorts the axonal topography of the brain, and decompression does more damage by allowing this distortion to spread further, resulting in a prognostically poor outcome. Reversing this CSF shift through cisternal drainage at atmospheric pressure detours the CSF from shifting into the paravascular spaces and the brain tissue, hence decreasing the intracranial pressure and preventing secondary axonal damage by preserving the neuronal topography at the same time.

Cisternostomy can thus be defined as a CSF let out microsurgical procedure to decrease intracranial pressure in moderate to severe brain injury. The pathophysiology of CSF shift edema forms the rationale of cisternostomy and its improved prognosis.

## Brain Cooling and Cleaning

### Brain as a Water Cooled and Cleaned System

The brain is a supercomputer which consumes about one-fifth of the blood supply of the body. While this makes the organ a center of huge levels of activity, it also needs a highly effective cleaning and cooling system. This cooling and cleaning system making use of the CSF in the cisterns and the Virchow Robin spaces as well as the pulsatility of the vessels traversing from the cisterns to the brain parenchyma is pure genius and if one understands this system, it would explain a whole lot of things like why we need to sleep, why does degenerative brain diseases happen after trauma or subarachnoid hemorrhage and how does "CSF shift edema" work.

We had proposed earlier that the brain is water cooled and water cleaned especially by the CSF.[5,9] These are independent pathways, the cooling pathway being continuous and using the paravascular spaces to convey cooled CSF to all around the brain, while the cleaning occurs in the night, or during sleep to be precise.

It is interesting that the cooling pathway makes use of the large air sinuses lined with mucosa as a heat loss mechanism. During breathing, the water from the wet mucosal linings evaporate fast just like a wet cloth cooling under a fan to lower the temperatures of the adjoining suprasellar cisterns (**Fig. 4.7**).

The cool CSF from the suprasellar cisterns is pumped into the brain through the paravascular Virchow Robin spaces accompanying the vessels (**Fig. 4.8**). These vessels provide the major blood supply to the basal brain structures and the pulsatility of these arteries traversing from the cisterns to the brain drives the cooled CSF from the suprasellar cisterns up into the brain through the Archimedes' screw principle.[10]

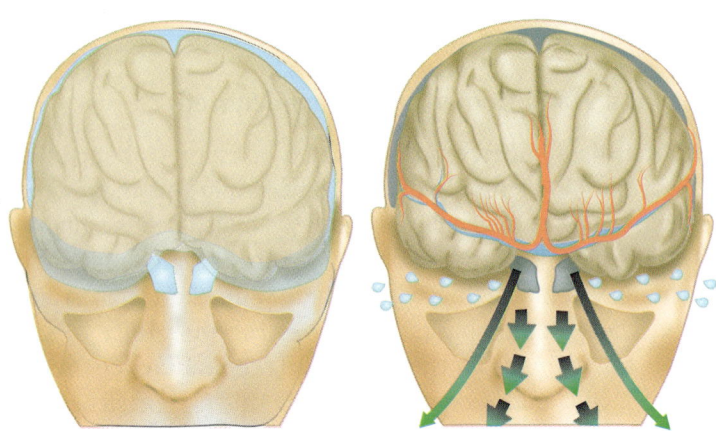

**Fig. 4.7** Brain cooling via breathing mechanism.

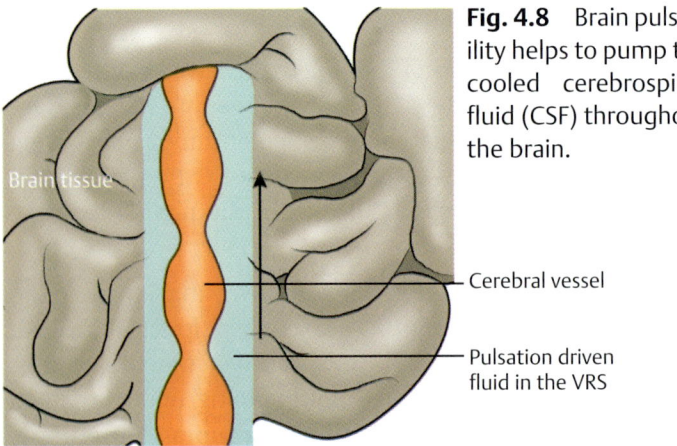

**Fig. 4.8** Brain pulsatility helps to pump the cooled cerebrospinal fluid (CSF) throughout the brain.

Brain tissue

Cerebral vessel

Pulsation driven fluid in the VRS

This is a passive event that is not dependent on the Aquaporin 4 channels and happens all through the day in a healthy individual.

In contrast, cleaning is a more active phenomena, which uses Aquaporin 4 gates to open in the night during sleep and create a mixture of CSF and brain interstitial fluid (ISF) to exchange nutrients and wastes to and from the brain.

This CSF–ISF mixing, and the fact that the daily turnover of CSF production and absorption is three- to four-fold of its volume in the brain unveils the many functions of the CSF other than providing buoyancy to the brain.

Understanding this intricate structure of the paravascular or, more precisely, the Virchow Robin spaces helps us understand the glymphatic system, which helps in explaining how the CSF communicating with the brain tissue in a dynamic fashion and integrating the laws of hydraulics, under pathological settings, changes the pressures and volumes of the fluid compartments to bring about gross edema and consequent brain shift, as seen in moderate to severe traumatic brain injuries.

So, it is evident that the glymphatic pathway does more than just nutrients exchange and waste removal. The glymphatic system has a role in the pathophysiology and management of some of the most common neurological and neurosurgical presentations. The CSF shift forms the rationale of cisternostomy—a micro-neurosurgical procedure for moderate to severe acute traumatic brain injury.

## The Paranasal Sinuses and the Bernoulli's Principle

The sinuses are strategically located such that the suprasellar cistern is in the center of the sinuses (**Fig. 4.9**). The cooling of the sinuses would lead to a cooling of the CSF in the suprasellar cisterns as well. In fact, it is interesting that deep breathing patterns like in Yoga would cool the sinuses more and cause more cooling of the brain. And single-sided breathing techniques like the *Anulom Vilom* may cool one side more selectively. As we breathe in and out, the airflow also enters the paranasal sinuses. However, since the entry points are small, the air entering the sinuses through these pores is at a higher velocity. This can be explained by the Bernoulli's principle[11] (**Fig. 4.9**).

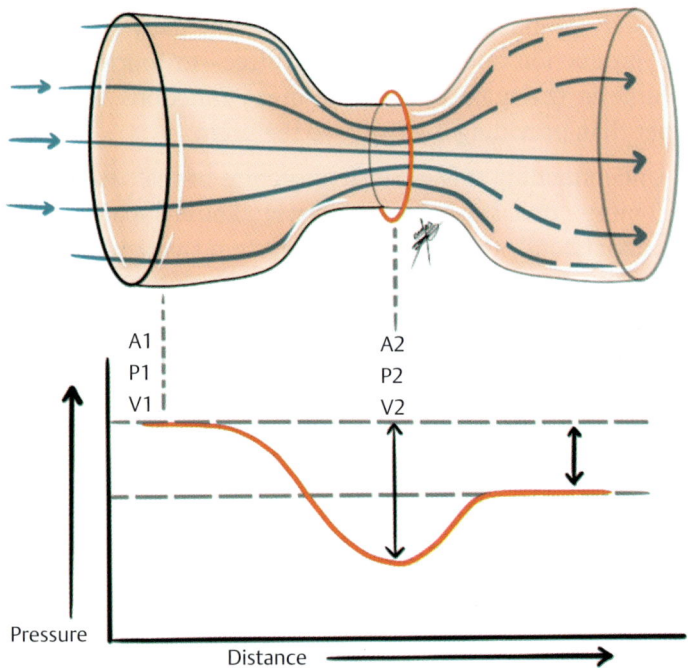

**Fig. 4.9** Simplified representation of the Bernoulli's principle. Image shows how a fluid going from a big tubular space to a smaller tubular space change the velocity and pressure of the fluid dramatically. A1, initial volume; P1, initial pressure; V1, initial velocity. Used with permission from Dr. Carlos Salvador Ovalle Torres.

## Conclusion

This high velocity of flow falling on the mucosa within the sinuses can lead to evaporation of the water content in the mucosa, and this would lead to the cooling of the sinuses because this evaporation would lead to loss of latent heat of evaporation (**Fig. 4.3**). Thus, all the sinuses are cooled in the same way that we cool ourselves by wearing a sweaty shirt and staying under the fan or just like how any other radiator works.

# References

1. Cherian I, Grasso G, Bernardo A, Munakomi S. Anatomy and physiology of cisternostomy. Chin J Traumatol 2016;19(1):7–10

2. Ziyal IM, Ozgen T, Sekhar LN, Ozcan OE, Cekirge S. Proposed classification of segments of the internal carotid artery: anatomical study with angiographical interpretation. Neurol Med Chir (Tokyo) 2005;45(4):184–190, discussion 190–191

3. Alfieri A, Jho HD. Endoscopic endonasal cavernous sinus surgery: an anatomic study. Neurosurgery 2001;48(4):827–836, discussion 836–837

4. Abdulrauf SI, Ashour AM, Marvin E, et al. Proposed clinical internal carotid artery classification system. [published correction appears in J Craniovertebr Junction Spine. 2017 Jan-Mar;8(1):84] J Craniovertebr Junction Spine 2016;7(3):161–170

5. Burhan H, Cherian I. Brain cooling and cleaning: a new perspective in cerebrospinal fluid (CSF) dynamics. In: Ambrosi PB, Ahmad R, Abdullahi A, Agrawal A, eds. New Insight into Cerebrovascular Diseases—An Updated Comprehensive Review. IntechOpen; February 21, 2020. DOI: 10.5772/intechopen.90484

6. Vijaywargiya M, Deopujari R, Athavale SA. Anatomical study of petrous and cavernous parts of internal carotid artery. Anat Cell Biol 2017;50(3):163–170

7. Labib MA, Prevedello DM, Carrau R, et al. A road map to the internal carotid artery in expanded endoscopic endonasal approaches to the ventral cranial base. Neurosurgery 2014;10(Suppl 3):448–471, discussion 471

8. Sameshima T, Mastronardi L, Friedman A, Fukushima T, eds. Middle fossa dissection for extended middle fossa and anterior petrosectomy approach. Fukushima's Microanatomy and Dissection of the Temporal Bone for Surgery of Acoustic Neuroma, and Petroclival Meningioma. 2nd ed. Raleigh: AF Neurovideo; 2007:51–83

9. Cherian I, Beltran M. A unified physical theory for CSF circulation, cooling and cleaning of the brain, sleep, and head injuries in degenerative cognitive disorders. In: Opris I, Casanova M, eds.

The Physics of the Mind and Brain Disorders. Springer Series in Cognitive and Neural Systems. Vol. 11. Cham: Springer; 2017:773–783

10. Cherian I, Beltran M, Kasper EM, Bhattarai B, Munokami S, Grasso G. Exploring the Virchow-Robin spaces function: a unified theory of brain diseases. Surg Neurol Int 2016;7(Suppl 26):S711–S714

11. Bernoulli's principle [Internet]. Wikipedia. Wikimedia Foundation; 2019. Available from: https://en.wikipedia.org/wiki/Bernoulli%27s_principle

# Radiological Indications in Cisternostomy

**5**

*Iype Cherian, Hira Burhan, and Ramdas Gidugu*

## Introduction

Cisternostomy is a time-dependent surgical approach to brain trauma. That said, it is important to identify the extent of intracranial injury and impending herniation. Radiological imaging provides this information and is helpful to determine the extent of injury, plan the surgical approach, and follow the prognosis postoperatively.

## Radiological Anatomy of Intracranial Lesions and Brain Herniation

Brain herniation is a consequence of the mass effects due to trauma, tumor, or cerebral abscess. A rise in the intracranial pressure leads to shift in the brain compartments giving rise to a series of anatomical distortions with clinical and radiological manifestations. The tentorium cerebelli separates the occipital lobes of cerebral hemispheres from the cerebellum. It is attached anteriorly to the clinoid processes of the sphenoid bone, anterolaterally to the petrous part of the temporal bone, and posterolaterally to the internal surface of occipital and the parietal bone. Superiomedially, tentorium cerebelli continues as falx cerebri, giving it a tent-like appearance. The tentorial notch or incisura is a semi-ovular opening through which the brain stem descends into the infratentorial compartment. The midbrain is located in the tentorial opening (incisura), and the uncus and para-hippocampal regions of the temporal lobe lie along the lateral margins of the tentorial incisura.

Transtentorial herniation occurs when the temporal lobe herniates down the tentorial notch. Bilateral descending tentorial herniations, which correspond to the axial pressure cone syndrome of Liliequist, occur mostly with frontal and central tumors, while lesions that are temporal or parietal in location tend to produce unilateral herniations or, herniations that are considerably larger on one side than on the other. Space-occupying lesions secondary to traumatic brain hemorrhages present with significant mass effects resulting in a mid-line shift and an obvious herniation as detected by obliterated basal cisterns on computed tomography (CT) imaging **(Fig. 5.1)**.

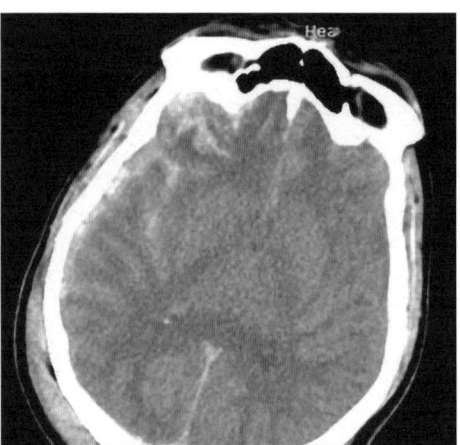

**Fig. 5.1** Obliterated cisterns on computed tomography (CT) imaging.

# The Cerebellopontine Angle Cistern and Impending Herniation

Supratentorial space-occupying lesions usually displace the anteromedial temporal lobe (uncus) into the tentorial incisura, a phenomenon called uncal herniation. Anatomically, the ambient cistern is located in both the supra- and infratentorial compartments demarcated by the tentorial incisura. As supratentorial pressure increases, uncal herniation happens, displacing the midbrain and the pons, causing widening of the ipsilateral infratentorial ambient cistern and narrowing or obliteration of the contralateral ambient cistern and cerebellopontine (CP) angle cistern.

Medial dislocation of uncus encroaches the lateral aspect of the suprasellar cistern indicating an impending tentorial herniation. In very early stages, the herniating anterior temporal lobe pushes the midbrain and the pons away, and occupies the ambient cistern resulting in the increased distance between the petrous bone and the pons, thereby widening the CP angle cistern on the same side as the expanding lesion (**Figs. 5.2** and **5.3**).

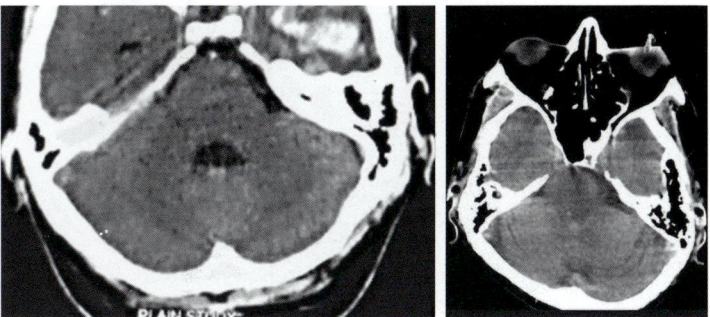

**Fig. 5.2** Identifying cerebellopontine (CP) angle cistern dilatation on computed tomography (CT) imaging.

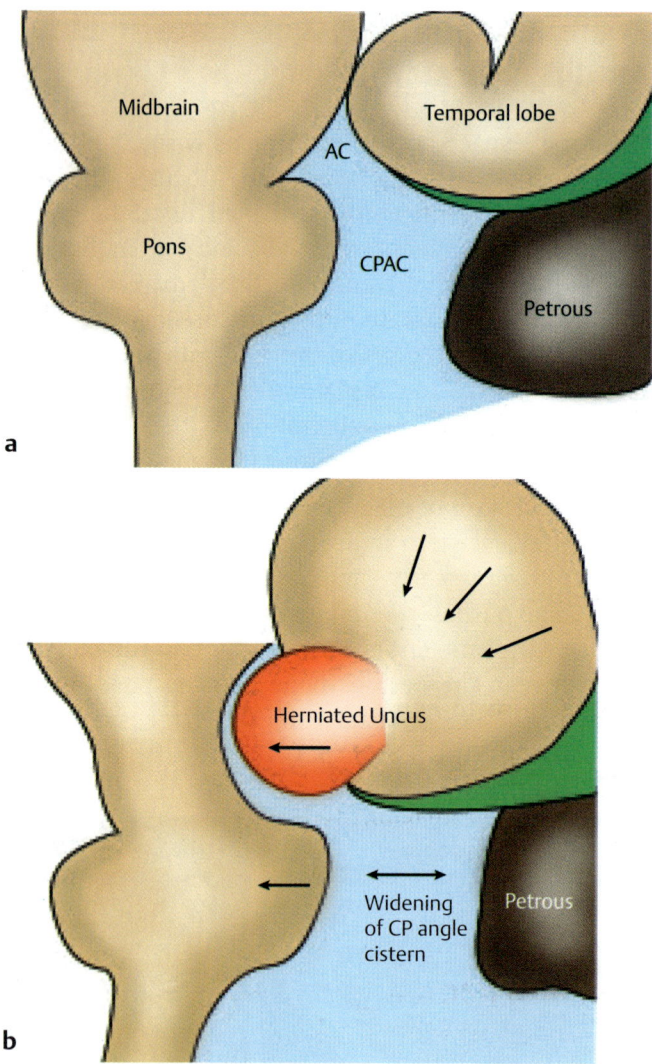

**Fig. 5.3** Sequel of widening of cerebellopontine (CP) angle cistern as the anterior temporal lobe begins to descend the tentorial notch. **(a)** Normal anatomy. **(b)** Descent of anterolateral temporal lobe (uncal herniation), pushing the midbrain and pons on the contralateral side. Notice widening of CP angle cistern. *(Continued)*

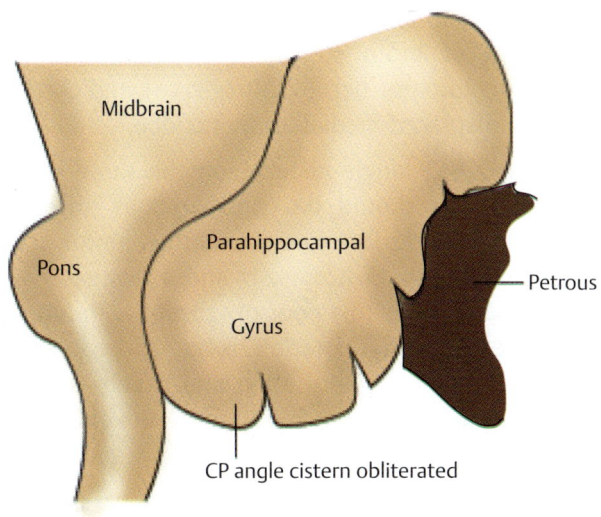

c

**Fig. 5.3** *(Continued)* **(c)** Transtentorial herniation and complete obliteration of CP angle cistern. AC: Ambient cistern; CPAC: Cerebellopontine angle cistern.

This gives rise to clinical manifestations of third nerve paresis and indicates increased intracranial pressure. These changes can be appreciated in very early on CT imaging or magnetic resonance imaging (MRI). Cranial CT is the mainstay of imaging and is preferred over MRI due to availability and speed of images.

## Correlating Radiological and Clinical Signs for Impending Herniation

It is of extreme importance to correlate the clinical signs with the radiological findings. The earliest sign of uncal herniation is the ipsilateral dilation of the pupil. A depressed state of consciousness is not a reliable early sign, but the patient may be confused or agitated. Other signs include contralateral or ipsilateral hemiparesis, resulting from compression or displacement of brain stem affecting ascending arousal pathways, oculomotor nerve (third nerve), and corticospinal tract by the displaced medial temporal lobe.

Widening of CP angle cisterns on the same side as the expanding lesion should be considered as an early sign of impending herniation. The presenting motor score is a significant predictor of prognosis and a decrease in motor score by 1 point leads to a poor prognosis. It should be clear that ipsilateral pupil dilatation is an early indication of impending or ongoing herniation and timely management using a cisternal drainage is required to prevent progression to a complete transtentorial herniation and thus poor prognosis.

Descending tentorial herniation has been further classified by Azambuja et al[1] into three subtypes: anterior, posterior, and complete herniations. In anterior herniation, only the uncus is involved and is herniated down into the ipsilateral crural cistern causing shifting and rotation of the brain stem. This anterior (uncal) herniation is the initial event in most cases of tentorial herniation, usually followed by herniation of more posteriorly located structures at a more advanced stage. A posterior herniation is present when the hippocampal gyrus (behind the uncus) has herniated down into the posterolateral part of the tentorial hiatus.

As the herniation progresses, it is possible that the uncus and para-hippocampal gyrus completely occupy and obliterate the entire ambient cistern and the CP angle cisterns.

The posterior herniations encroach upon the lateral part of the quadrigeminal plate cistern and will cause a displacement, rotation, and compression of the brain stem. When both anterior and posterior herniations are present and join each other, the result is a complete herniation **(Fig. 5.4)**.

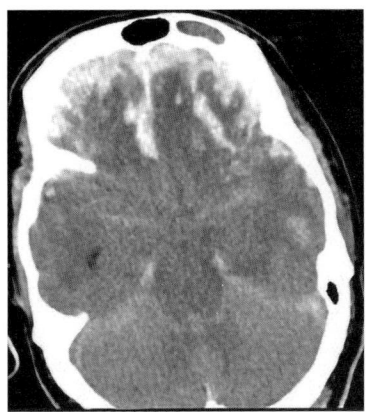

**Fig. 5.4** Complete herniation.

As this progression happens, the brain stem is compressed as well as undergoes torsion, resulting in rapid clinical deterioration—the conscious state may deteriorate to a deep coma. The consequent clinical findings would start with a constriction and then dilatation of the ipsilateral pupil due to oculomotor nerve compression; however, para-hippocampal gyrus herniation, causing further compression and torsion of the brain stem, would worsen the picture and clinical deterioration would result, with bad prognosis.

Bilateral dilated pupils and a decreased Glasgow coma scale (GCS) with a motor score of 3 define the progression to an advanced stage of herniation with the para-hippocampal gyrus involvement, which causes effacement of cisternal spaces at the tentorial level and compressing of the contralateral anterior cerebral peduncle (crus cerebri) against the tentorium, resulting in ipsilateral hemiparesis (Kernohan's false localizing sign). Time is of the essence in such pathologies and early surgical intervention might result in a better prognosis.

The herniation of para-hippocampal gyrus should not however be misinterpreted as a posterior fossa tumor on radiological imaging. These findings, consistent with the preoperative CT scans in more severe patients, are often accompanied by complete third nerve palsy and follow a poorer response in clinical status.

## Time is Essence!

One important factor in management of cerebral herniation is the time lapsed before presenting to the emergency department (ED). In early signs of brain injury, a widened CP angle cistern can be well appreciated in the images obtained upon arrival. The initial events of anterior temporal lobe herniation present with a GCS score of above 8 and a motor score of 5 and 4 only in some patients, with unilateral (ipsilateral) pupil dilation and widened CP angle cistern.

## Indicators of Good Prognosis

- GCS >8 (motor score 4–5).
- Ipsilateral pupil dilation.
- CP angle widening.

This determines a good prognostic value as shown by our postoperative outcomes. In a later sequel, transtentorial herniation may cause ipsilateral cerebral infarction due to occlusion of the posterior cerebral artery and the Duret hemorrhage, which typically occurs in the ventral and paramedian midbrain/pons following rapid downward herniation.

## Other Signs of Uncal Herniation on CT

- Shift of mesencephalon.
- Obliteration of suprasellar cisterns.

- Aqueductal compression.
- Hydrocephalus.
- Descending tentorial herniation (DTH).

The magnitude of rise in intracranial pressure secondary to traumatic brain injury can be observed by the edematous brain peroperatively. In patients presenting with signs of impending herniations as identified by widened CP angle cisterns on the same side as the expanding lesion, timely cisternostomy to let out cerebrospinal fluid from the basal cisterns rapidly decreases cerebral edema, getting the brain lax enough for bone flap re-apposition at the end of the procedure. This timely intervention further prevents progression to herniation of the edematous brain into an artificial cavity, stretching of axons and neural structures and probably high intraparenchymal pressure despite decrease in intracranial pressure which later would contribute to a higher morbidity and vegetative patient outcome otherwise seen in traditional decompressive hemicraniectomy.

## Conclusion

Cisternostomy is a relatively new treatment for head injuries, which needs proactive intervention like decompressive hemicraniectomy. Therefore, subtle radiological signs and the understanding of relative clinical symptoms are important. This has been discussed in this chapter which would be useful to young neurosurgeons who will venture in this practice.

## Reference

1. Azambuja N, Lindgren E, Sjogren SE. Tentorial herniations. II. Pneumography. Acta Radiol 1956;46(1-2):224–231

# 6

# Cisternostomy— How I Do It

*Iype Cherian and J.K.B.C. Parthiban*

## Introduction

Performing cisternostomy requires intricate surgical skills for instrument handling and complex maneuvers. For young neurosurgeons cisternostomy has a steep learning curve requiring training and mentorship from more experienced neurosurgeons who are performing this routinely. This chapter outlines the surgical expertise from two senior neurosurgeons from India who describe their "How I do it" for teaching and learning purposes.

## How I Do It by Iype Cherian

### Introduction

The author started the technique of cisternostomy for severe head trauma circa 2007, and this was an act of serendipity. What happened in essence was that he managed a severe head trauma like he would do a bad grade aneurysm. In bad grade aneurysms, one would try and open the cisterns as early as possible. The sylvian fissure dissection is not an option here since the brain is swollen.

One needs to get into the optico-carotid, caroticooculomotor cistern and then open the membrane of Liliequist. And for this a very basal approach is required with very generous drilling of the sphenoid, the orbital roof in an extradural manner, and sometimes the anterior clinoid also needs to be taken in an extradural fashion.

## Brain Unlocking Maneuvers

The three "unlocking" planes, namely, sagittal, axial, and intradural oblique unlocking (sylvian dissection), are used to access the base of the brain. The sagittal unlocking is about drilling the sphenoid ridge and the orbital roof and making a direct access into the optic nerve and carotid to open the anterior cisterns.

Axial unlocking is about peeling off the temporal lobe from the cavernous sinus and then having an access to the interpeduncular cistern. Oblique intradural unlocking (sylvian dissection) is the more commonly used one; however, it cannot be used in a tight brain like in trauma.

## Positioning

The author positions the patient on a horse shoe with the body elevated 15 degrees, the head extended and turned about 20 degrees to the opposite side. His craniotomy side is determined by the subdural and midline shift, extensive contusions, or the right side (in that order).

## Craniotomy

The author does a frontotemporal craniotomy which is much smaller than the one used for decompression (**Fig. 6.1**). He tries and reach the temporal base flush and also drills the sphenoid base as much as possible.

Generous drilling of the sphenoid allows for visualization of the orbito-meningeal band (OMB), which comes between the frontal and temporal lobe. Dissecting the OMB at high resolution allows you to reach a plane that enables the

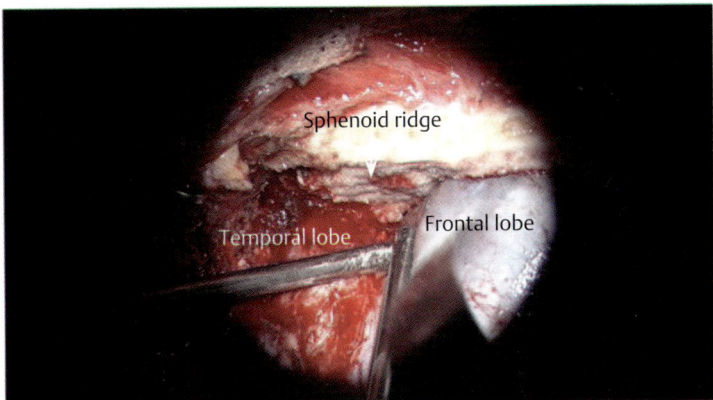

**Fig. 6.1** Frontotemporal craniotomy and ongoing removal of the sphenoid ridge.

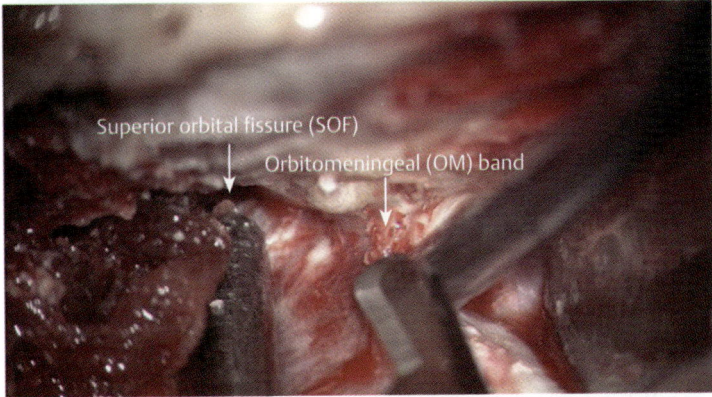

**Fig. 6.2** Sharp cutting of the orbito-meningeal (OM) band under high magnification.

peeling of the temporal dura off the cavernous sinus without any bleeding (**Fig. 6.2**).

Care needs to be taken not to compromise the true cavernous membrane, which can result in significant bleeding. For minor bleedings, the author prefers to use surgicels over fibrin glue as the later can result in cavernous sinus thrombosis making the brain more tense. These are the important steps toward a bloodless extradural lateralization of the temporal lobe **(Fig. 6.3)**.

Dissecting the OMB toward the frontal lobe provides a window for anterior clinoidectomy, if needed **(Fig. 6.4)**.

The author also dissects the subfrontal dura in an extradural fashion and shave off the orbital roof in an

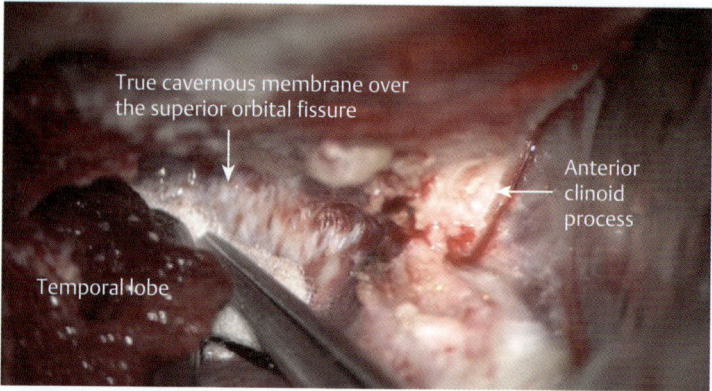

**Fig. 6.3** Peeling of superior orbital fissure (SOF) dura preserving the true cavernous membrane.

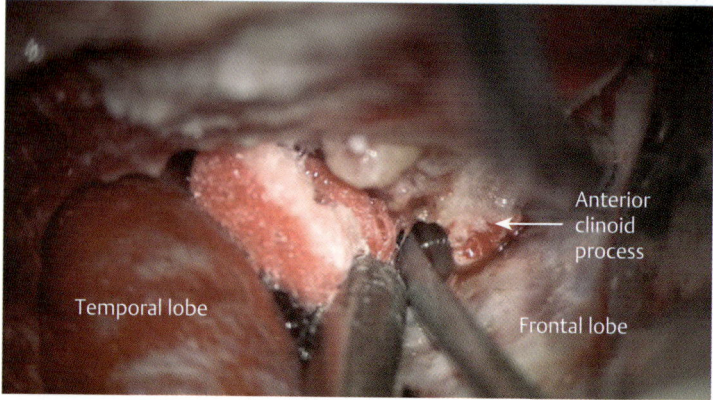

**Fig. 6.4** Uncovering the anterior clinoid by dissecting the orbito-meningeal (OM) band on the frontal side.

extradural fashion to facilitate easy entry into the optico-carotid and lateral carotid cisterns. It is to be noted that the amount of bone removed can be up to 30 mL in the base and this is something that would get the brain to be a little bit more lax than the usual decompressive hemicraniectomies.

## Dural Opening

As opposed to the standard "C"-shaped opening, a basal dural opening is performed in cisternostomy (**Fig. 6.5**). The dural opening is made as basal as possible to facilitate a direct access to the cisterns and prevent the brain herniation. However, with all these measures, it is not uncommon that the frontal brain herniates to some extent into the operative field till one can open the optico-carotid and lateral carotid cisterns.

## Cisternal Opening

Once the dura is opened, a wide brain retractor is put in below the frontal lobe and it is retracted to access the optic and the carotid (**Fig. 6.6**).

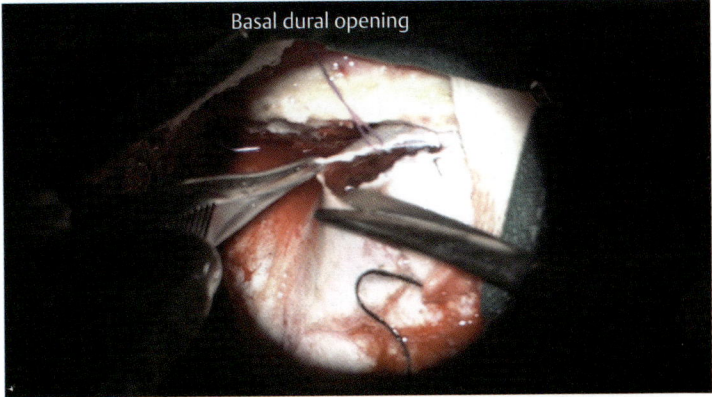

**Fig. 6.5** Basal dural opening.

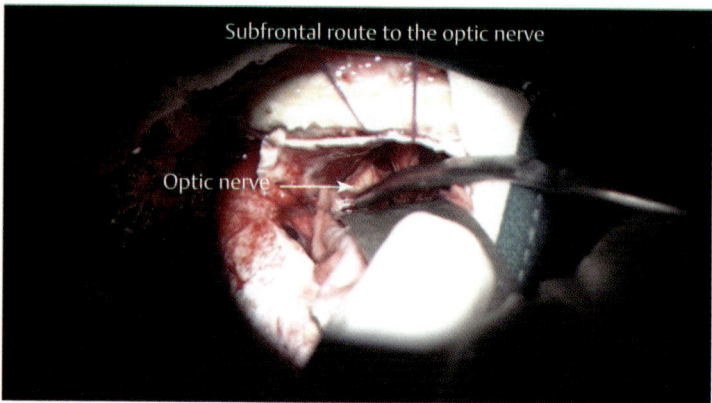

**Fig. 6.6** Subfrontal route is one of the first and fast steps done in an exceedingly tight brain.

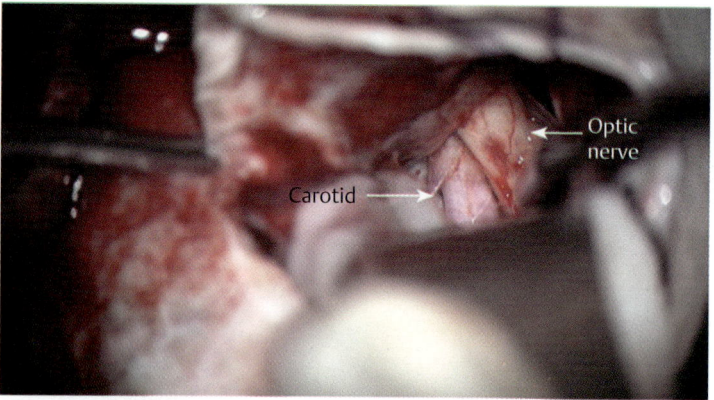

**Fig. 6.7** Exposing the optico-carotid window.

Once the cisterns associated with these structures are opened, good irrigation is done and the blood is cleared from these cisterns (**Fig. 6.7**).

After this, depending on whether the optico-carotid cistern or the lateral carotid cistern is easier to dissect and is larger, the membrane of Liliequist is opened through either of them (**Fig. 6.8**).

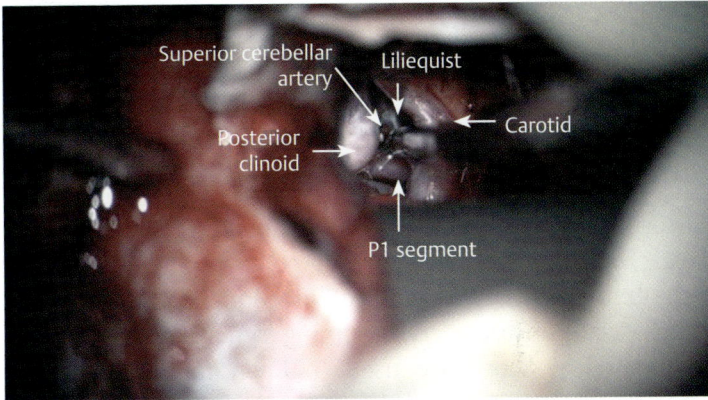

**Fig. 6.8** Dissection of membrane of Liliequist to expose P1 and superior cerebellar artery.

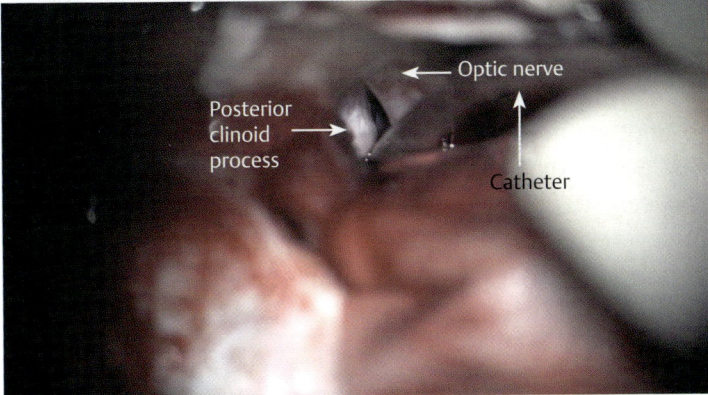

**Fig. 6.9** Insertion of a number 8 feeding tube/EVD tube through lateral carotid window.

A drainage tube is put into the prepontine cistern and continuous irrigation is carried out till the closure is done (**Fig. 6.9**).

Dura is left open and large surgicels are put above the dura. The bone is kept back as a free flap. Closure is done in layers.

## "How I Do It"—Negotiating Basal Cisterns in Cisternostomy Procedure by J.K.B.C. Parthiban

### Introduction

Cisternostomy is nothing but opening of arachnoid layers of the cisterns to let out cerebrospinal fluid (CSF) and to make way for surgical procedures. But in recent times "cisternostomy" is becoming synonymous with the microsurgical procedure used to open up basal cisterns and let out CSF in severe head trauma to reduce cerebral edema. Although opening the cisterns in nontraumatic and nonsubarachnoid hemorrhagic conditions like aneurysms are easier under microsurgical visualization, it is not so in conditions where there are severe cerebral edema and significant subarachnoid hemorrhage (SAH). The art of negotiating in the cisterns to reach from one compartment to another needs certain extra skill among neurosurgeons that need to be learned. Once the techniques are understood it is easy to perform cisternostomy in rough conditions like in severe head injury. This chapter will try to explain the important steps involved in a simple format.

### Complete Cisternostomy

Cisternostomy in head injury patients with significant cerebral edema is aimed to reduce the intracranial pressure by letting out CSF that is locked up in basal cisterns due to SAH. To achieve satisfactory result CSF should be let out from both supra- and infratentorial cisterns since SAH can be diffuse and present in both compartments. The Liliequist membrane divides them by two layers, diencephalic layer and mesencephalic layer, and extends between the third nerves on both side and beyond. Opening the Liliequist membrane through the supratentorial cisterns (carotid cisterns) is essential to enter into infratentorial cistern (prepontine). This will let out CSF from infratentorial cistern, and washing of SAH blood with saline can be performed to further improve CSF let out. While CSF is let out significant amount of subarachnoid blood is also washed out from the cisterns. Hence, a "complete cisternostomy" is defined as a procedure that include opening of both supra- and infratentorial cisterns by opening Liliequist membrane and washing out blood while letting out CSF (**Fig. 6.10**). Any procedure that falls short of this is considered as "partial or incomplete cisternostomy."

## Position and Craniotomy

For a successful cisternostomy, the head should be positioned as we do in aneurysm surgery—well extended, zygoma at the top in pterional approach through a fronto-temporoparietal (FTP) craniotomy and tip of the nose at top for subfrontal approach through a bifrontal craniotomy (**Fig. 6.11**). It is vital to fix the head with a three-pin head fixator in order to

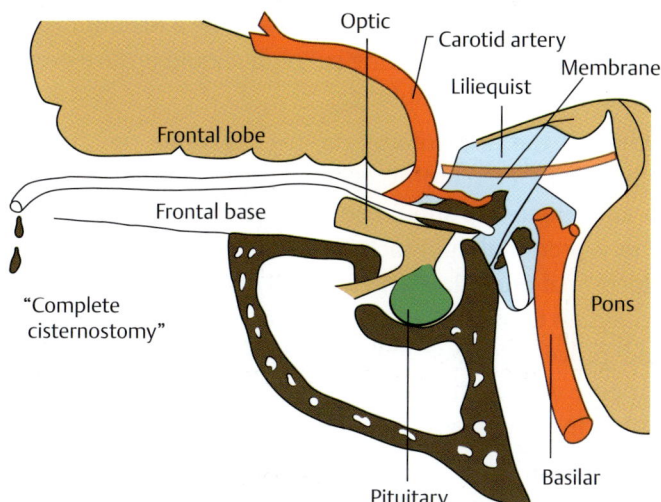

**Fig. 6.10** Complete cisternostomy.

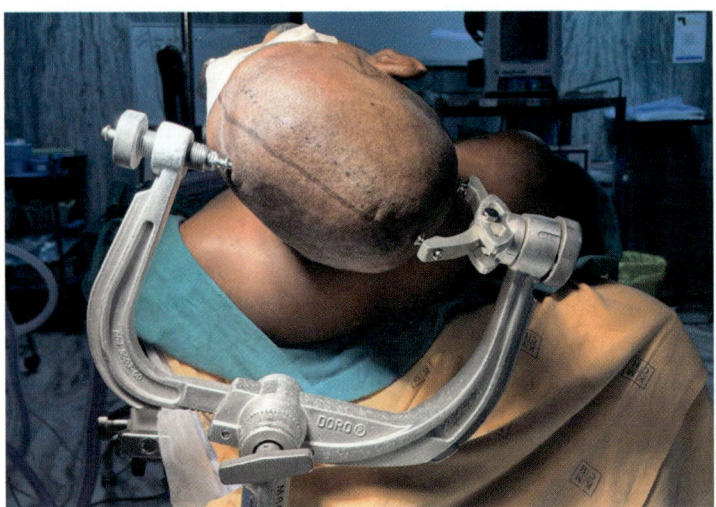

**Fig. 6.11** Head fixed with three-pin system.

secure the position during the surgical procedure. Surgeons who fail to use the fixators and position the head over head ring will never get the right trajectory since the head will move during rotating the bone flap. Repositioning will be difficult and aim of reaching cisterns will be a distant task all together. Hence, the operating surgeon should ensure proper head fixation before scrubbing.

Whether the craniotomy is big as done in classical decompressive craniotomy or small as needed, the base of the cranial bone flap should be flush at frontal and temporal base in a pterional approach or at both side of frontal base in a bicoronal bone flap. The lesser wing of sphenoid should be drilled up to anterior clinoid process. Removal of anterior clinoid process further improves easiness of reaching the optic nerve. Although it is not mandatory in all cases, but it is indicated in very severe cerebral edema. Dura thus exposed is dissected well and the orbitomeningeal bands be separated from its attachment to bony anatomy. This step releases the dura and surfaces it on par with anterior cranial base dura and temporal base dura, thus unlocking the frontal and temporal lobes (**Fig. 6.12a–c**). Removal of bones up to the base of frontal and temporal fossae and entire lesser wing of sphenoid is the key step for reaching the basal cisterns. Surgeons who fail to achieve the above-mentioned head positioning and bone work can never achieve satisfactory cisternostomy.

## Approach

In normal conditions surgical approach to optico-carotid cistern is simple, when the head is positioned with the neck extended and dropped toward floor as in all aneurysm surgeries; the gravitational retraction of frontal lobe allows easy retraction, exposing the arachnoid layer over the optic nerve. Incising the arachnoid opens the cisterns and CSF will flow out; dissection around carotids and optic nerve is easy. Depending on the anatomy it is easy to negotiate blunt and sharp micro instruments like microscissors through the cisterns at depth. Hence, reaching the Liliequist through carotico-optic and lateral carotid cisterns is much easier in normal circumstances. In SAH with no significant mass effect this can be appreciated. However, the scenario in traumatic brain edema is completely different.

In a tight brain reaching the optico-carotid (OC) cistern is a challenge and needs technical expertise that can be mastered in short time. The best and short way to reach OC cistern is to perform excision of lesser wing of sphenoid by drilling the bone as close to anterior clinoid process as possible and dissecting the dura from frontotemporal base by releasing orbito-meningeal band as mentioned earlier. This one step makes the procedure easy since the area of basifrontal lobe retraction is minimal and distance between the surgeon and OC cistern becomes much shorter in pterional approach when compared to the subfronal approach and when lesser wing sphenoid ridge was not removed in a pterional approach.

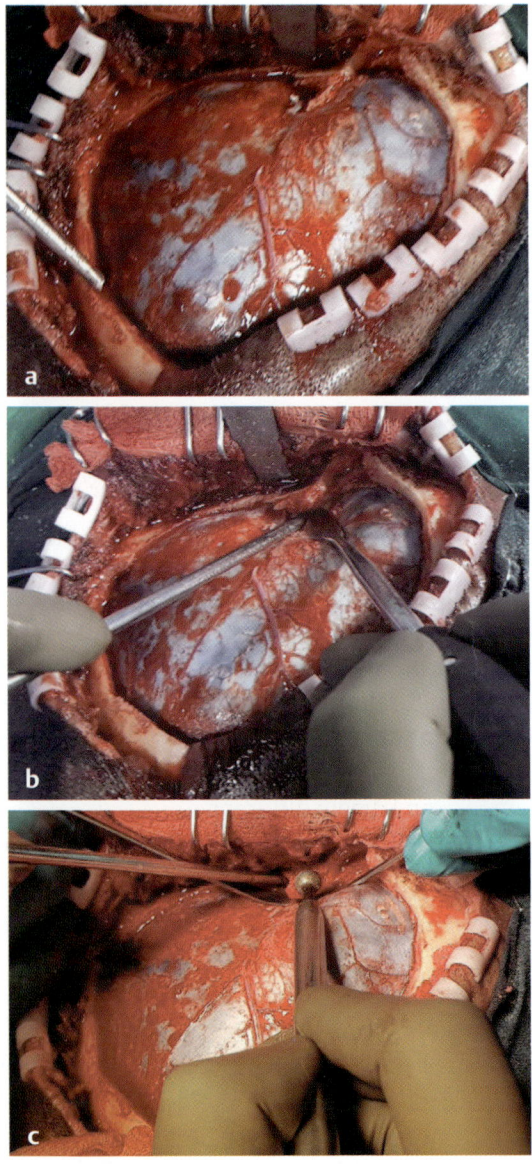

**Fig. 6.12** **(a)** Large craniotomy. **(b)** Lesser wing sphenoid exposed. **(c)** Drilling of Lesser wing sphenoid.

Retracting the edematous frontal lobe needs extra effort and saline-soaked cotton patties should be used over the frontal base while the lobe is being retracted with suction tube itself. Ideally, we should "crawl" over the frontal base along with cotton patties until we reach the optic nerve. Intermittent retraction is sufficient, and the tense brain tends to push the retractor cotton patties. Once the optic nerve is reached, retractor blade can, if needed, now be replaced over the cotton patties. I usually avoid using metal retractors. Contused basifrontal lobe with pial breach tends to pulp out during retraction, overflowing around the retractor blade and should be removed. Removal of large hematomas and contusion does relax the lobe and facilitate easy retraction.

## Arachnoid Dissection

Cisternostomy is all about arachnoid dissection and strictly a microsurgical procedure. Arachnoid layer over the optic nerve should be teased, cut, and opened, dissecting around the nerve on both sides. Carotid artery seen laterally is usually very close to the optic nerve and needs to be dissected away from the optic nerve to create the corridor. Further dissection and arachnoid teasing between the nerve and artery can lead to Liliequist membrane (**Fig. 6.13a, b**). The multilayered membrane with septae needs to be teased out to further progress dissection to infratentorial compartment visualizing basilar artery and few perforators on the way (**Fig. 6.14a**). The prepontine cistern thus opens, with carotid cisterns establishing a communication between supra- and infratentorial CSF compartments. Two important structures to be observed during this dissection are the pituitary stalk and posterior crinoid process. A large posterior clinoid may obstruct the route and the surgeon can either go lateral to carotids or rarely may need to excise the clinoid, which needs extraordinary surgical skill.

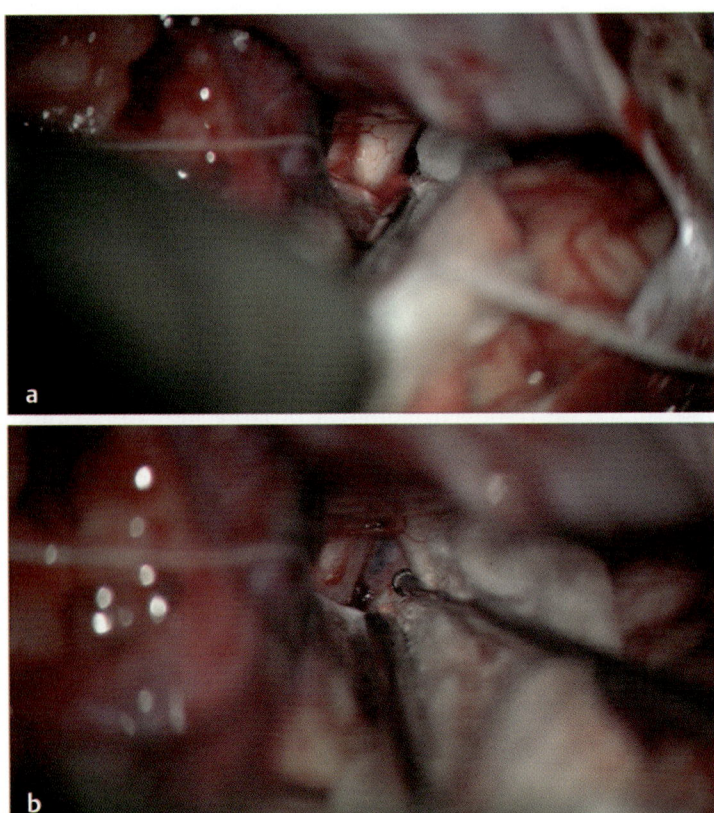

**Fig. 6.13** **(a)** Optico-carotid corridor. **(b)** Liliequist membrane.

Wide arachnoid dissection allows CSF and blood to get washed out systematically and the more the CSF is let out the more the brain becomes lax. Arachnoid dissection lateral to carotids and chiasm provides more lateral approach to prepontine cistern. We also open inter-optic cisterns to let out more and more CSF. Continuous saline wash helps in washing out bloody CSF and relaxes the brain further that can be appreciated by the easiness of dissection and less force needed for retraction.

## Cisternostomy Drain Tube

Although the author used ventricular end of regular shunt tubes in the initial period, he switched over to the external ventricular drainage (EVD) tubes due to its wide bore and less slippery nature. The tip of the tube should be gently inserted through the rent in Liliequist membrane into the prepontine cistern (**Fig. 6.14b**). Often, there is a tendency to insert the tube further in order to secure the tip perfectly in the desired site but end up placing much deeper on the cistern even up to

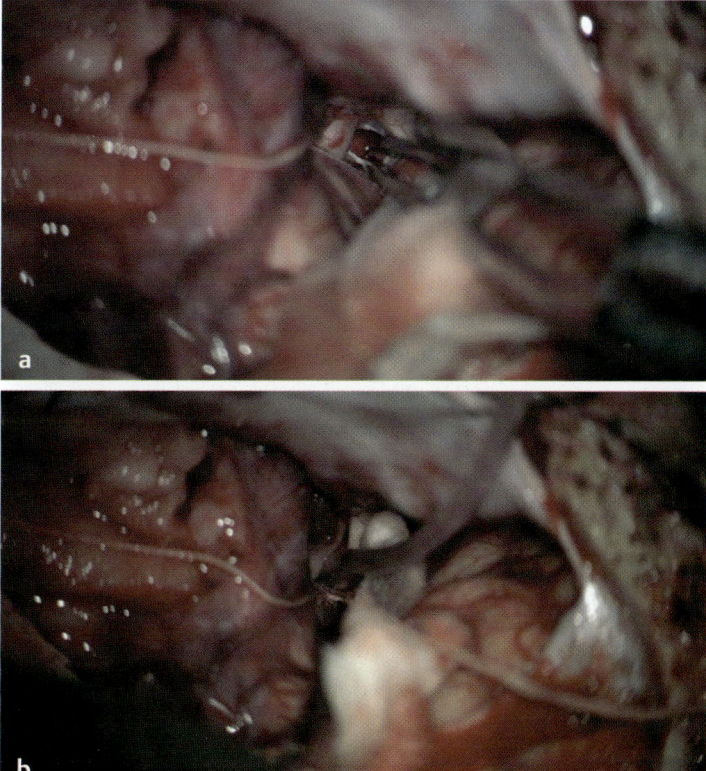

**Fig. 6.14** **(a)** Liliequist membrane opened. **(b)** Cisternal drain placed.

cerebellopontine cistern and the tip seen touching the pons and piercing the anterior surface by a few millimeters. This is usually detected in follow-up CT scans. In this situation it can repositioned by gently pulling out as much as it is needed. The cisternostomy tube is brought out through a separate stab wound in the scalp beyond the incision and secured well to the scalp to avoid migration and pullout while performing postoperative care. The author noticed approximately 9-cm length of the tube from prepontine to the calvarium in Indian patients and this observation helps in proper positioning of the tip. After the surgical procedure the tube is connected to the bag and the bag is placed at the same level as the head position. We usually keep it at a lower level on day 1 postoperatively to check the flow of CSF and later bring it to the same level.

Normally 150 to 200 cc of CSF is collected in the bag every 24 hours. However, we have noticed large volume of 250 cc and more on few occasions. Overflow of CSF is detrimental and in these situations we either increase the height of the collecting bag or close the flow and release it intermittently to achieve around 200 cc. Occasionally CSF drains well initially and later stops abruptly. This occurs usually due to a block in the tube that may need to be flushed with saline using 1-cc syringe gently and rotating the tube. This maneuver usually opens the tube and CSF starts draining well.

Cisternostomy tube can be kept in place for 5 to 7 days depending on the need and we tend to keep it for longer days. We also have used midstream CSF for microbiology lab testing when meningitis is suspected. Antibiotics in general and in specific according to results is routine in our practice while keeping the tube. Improvement in clinical status, radiological improvement, and laboratory results are taken into account before removing the cisternostomy tube. Cessation of CSF flow and worsening or nonimprovement of clinical status indicates poor prognosis.

# Conclusion: Important Steps for Successful Complete Cisternostomy

- Fix the head with three-pin fixator.
- Position the head with zygoma on top for pterional approach and nose for subfrontal approach.
- Drill lesser wing sphenoid liberally.
- Microsurgical technique to negotiate through the cisterns beyond Liliequist membrane.
- Proper positioning and securing of cisternostomy drain.

# 7
# Perspective, Long-Term, Experience, and Results

## 7A Perspectives about Cisternostomy
*Yonghong Wang*

## Introduction of Cisternostomy

Cisternostomy is a modern microsurgical treatment of head injury which provides a more physiological approach in the management of brain swelling by opening intracranial basal cisterns (the optic chiasmatic cistern, carotid cistern, and prepontine cistern). By doing cisternostomy in a traumatized swollen brain, there is a backward movement of the cerebrospinal fluid (CSF) to the various cisterns through the Virchow-Robin spaces. By inserting a drainage tube in the cisterns (prepontine cistern) after surgery to continuously drain CSF (5–7 days), there is a positive potential to control intracranial pressure (ICP) effectively. The brain edema reduces which in turn decreases secondary brain damage. It also helps in lowering the rates of vasospasm and hydrocephalus and improves the clinical prognosis of severe brain injury.

This technique is an advance in neurocritical surgery. Cisternostomy represents a valuable option for the treatment of choice in neurocritical surgery. Basal cisternal drainage not only effectively controls ICP but also reduces brain damage secondary to brain edema.

## The Pathophysiology of Basal Cisternostomy

The key to the effective evaluation of cisternostomy is a thorough understanding of the pathophysiological mechanism and, more so, the discovery of the glymphatic system, which has revolutionized our perception of interstitial waste clearance and CSF circulation in the brain.

The most recent theory and viewpoint regarding the third circulation involve the production of CSF in the choroid plexus and locations outside the choroid, the flow of CSF through the ventricles into the subarachnoid space, the significance of CSF entering the glymphatic system in facilitating brain clearance and maintaining homeostasis, and the elimination of CSF and brain extracellular fluid (ECF) through the lymphatic vessels of the dura mater, perineuronal spaces, parasagittal spaces, and arachnoid granulations. The absence of smooth muscle in the meningeal lymphatic vasculature renders it particularly susceptible to variations in pressure and brain edema within the rigid skull structure. Traumatic brain injury (TBI) leads to compromised drainage of meningeal lymphatic vessels and elevated ICP, which can hinder the drainage function of meningeal lymphatics and impact glymphatic system operation. By preventing the sudden increase in ICP following TBI, there may be an opportunity to address the ongoing dysfunction of both the glymphatic and lymphatic systems post brain injury.

The glymphatic system aids in the conveyance of interstitial fluid (ISF) to the CSF adjacent to the brain, while the lymphatic system absorbs CSF/ISF for subsequent conveyance to the periphery. The meningeal lymphatics potentially serve as a crucial pathway for draining CSF into the peripheral blood. Recent studies have shown that the efficacy of glymphatics, involving paravascular CSF influx and ISF efflux of macromolecules, is influenced by the function of meningeal lymphatics.

The involvement of the glymphatic system in regulating brain swelling and CSF dynamics in various neurosurgical conditions is evident, with the AQP4 channels playing a central role in this complex system. These investigations collectively propose that abnormalities within the glymphatic system could not only contribute to the advancement of neurosurgical disorders but also offer a route for therapeutic interventions through restoration. Cisternostomy, as one of these pathways, suggests that drainage of basal cisterns post subarachnoid hemorrhage (SAH) could enhance patient outcomes by aiding in CSF clearance, thereby reducing the risk of secondary injuries and unfavorable prognoses at the 6-month mark. Given that cerebral edema may primarily consist of CSF, the introduction of drainage mechanisms could potentially alleviate the progression of edema.

Brain tissue damage and edema and elevated ICP may exacerbate the patients' condition by inducing subsequent brain injury and swiftly compromising the meningeal lymphatic system's clearance function as well as the glymphatic system's capacity for CSF and ISF exchange. The cisternostomy procedure, currently employed during the acute phase of severe TBI to mitigate ICP via an intracranial basal cistern stoma and cistern CSF drainage, serves to avert brain edema and secondary damage. Post-TBI intracerebral hemorrhage contributes to glymphatic system impairment, leading to the entry of blood-derived metabolites into the cistern.

The repercussions of TBI outcomes are notably influenced by the presence of brain edema.

# Clearance Pathway of Brain Edema Fluid

Within the tissue, the pressure gradients arise which serve as the primary driving forces behind the dispersion of edema fluid. A notable discrepancy in ISF pressure (IFP) is observed between the edema region and the pressures in the CSF and normal brain tissue. The elevation of IFP appears to trigger the expansion of the extracellular space (ECS). An important mechanism for resolving vasogenic brain edema involves the entry of edema fluid into the CSF. The production of ISF in the normal brain likely occurs at the capillary–glial complex, with subsequent flow through low-resistance pathways (perivascular spaces) into the CSF. Perivascular spaces may act as conduits for fluid interchange between the brain and CSF. In instances of vasogenic brain edema following brain injury, there is a significant enlargement of the ECS. These expanded spaces potentially offer a route for the movement of edema fluid. The clearance of edema fluid into the CSF appears to be linked to the hydrostatic pressure gradient between the IFP in the edematous tissue and the CSF pressure (CSFP). Alterations in CSFP can directly impact the volume and speed of this clearance process. Therefore, a reduction in CSFP could promote edema fluid clearance by augmenting this pressure gradient, while an increase in CSFP might have the opposite effect. Current treatments such as hypertonic saline, mannitol, and decompressive craniectomy, although effective in reducing intracranial hypertension, have uncertain effects on outcomes, underscoring the delicate balance between adaptive and pathological swelling. Future strategies for treating cerebral edema post-TBI may necessitate targeted interventions based on the underlying pathophysiology, focusing on enhancing the clearance of edema fluid at the tissue–ventricular CSF interface. A transformative shift in approach is emerging—basal cisternal drainage.

## The Role of Basal Cistern Drainage

The following points describe the role of basal cistern drainage:

- It can reduce ICP and brain edema effectively.
- It can relieve cerebral vasospasm, relieve local acidosis, and improve prognosis.
- It is helpful to reduce the incidence of traumatic hydrocephalus.
- It can relieve brain stem compression.
- It can replace ventricular puncture drainage or repeated lumbar puncture drainage of bloody CSF.

## Conclusion

Cisternostomy is a surgical procedure utilized for the purpose of managing ICP and decreasing brain edema. Specifically, cisternostomy of the basal cisterns is a method deemed suitable for treating certain patients suffering from various conditions such as TBI, cerebral hemorrhage, cerebral infarction, aneurysmal SAH, arachnoid cyst, and large brain tumors that may develop significant brain edema post-surgery. Moreover, cisternostomy presents itself as a viable option compared to decompressive craniectomy (DC) due to its lower associated costs, reduced morbidity, and diminished mortality rates, as it involves a single neurosurgical intervention.

# Perspectives of Cisternostomy from Iraq

## 7B

*Ahmed Muthana, Osman Elamin, Fatimah O. Ahmed, and Samer S. Hoz*

## Introduction

In low- and middle-income countries, cisternostomy has emerged as a significant advancement in the field of neurotraumatology. This technique is employed for managing posttraumatic brain swelling in cases of traumatic brain injury (TBI) and acute intraoperative brain swelling during specific neurosurgical procedures such as intracerebral hemorrhage (ICH). The present chapter presents two cases from Iraq that were treated with cisternostomy—one involving ICH and the other TBI. Furthermore, the chapter elaborates on the categorization of cisternostomy according to its mechanism and clinical indications.

Cisternostomy is a novel approach that integrates the skill sets of skull base and microvascular surgery to manage brain edema and herniation resulting from elevated intracranial pressure.[1,2] This technique involves the precise microsurgical creation of openings in the basal cisterns, facilitating the equalization of cisternal pressure with atmospheric pressure. As a result, cerebrospinal fluid (CSF) can transfer from the brain tissue to the basal cisterns, ultimately easing brain tension.[3]

In cases of TBI, the primary utilization of cisternostomy can be seen in TBI. This procedure, when combined with decompressive craniectomy (DC), aims to counteract the harmful progression that leads to posttraumatic brain swelling. It serves as a last resort in the management of medically resistant severe TBI.[4,5] Furthermore, cisternostomy can be applied to address sudden instances of "brain swelling" that may arise during various neurosurgical procedures, such as those involving aneurysms, tumors, or ICH.[4,6] The CSF produced from cisterns interacts with brain tissue through Virchow-Robin spaces, as indicated by investigations conducted on glymphatics.[7,8]

In low- and middle-income countries (LMICs) with limited resources, cisternostomy emerges as a rare development in the field of neurotraumatology.[9] The popularity of cisternostomy has significantly increased in various LMICs over the last 8 years, extending from its place of origin, Nepal, to neurosurgical centers in countries such as China, Egypt, Brazil, India, Iran, and Iraq, due to its reduced risks and cost-effectiveness. Nonetheless, cisternostomy remains a complex microsurgical procedure, and only a limited number of neurosurgeons in LMICs have the necessary skills and equipment to perform it safely.[10] The availability of microscopes through initiatives like fellowships and manufacturing of affordable microscopes is crucial for the progress of cisternostomy.[11]

In this section, the authors recount their involvement with cisternostomy in one of the LMICs, Iraq.

Initially, the authors showcased two cases effectively managed through cisternostomy: one related to a TBI scenario and the other involving an ICH event. Subsequently, they expound upon two categorization systems of cisternostomy grounded on the mode of operation and specific indications.

# Illustrative Cases

## Case 1: Cisternostomy in Acute TBI

A 3-year-old girl arrived at the emergency room after falling from a height of 6 meters, with a Glasgow Coma Scale score of 10 out of 15 (E2M5V3). Initial assessments, including a quick history and examination, were conducted, and intravenous (IV) access was established for the administration of isotonic IV fluids. Upon examination, it was noted that the patient had an irregular 8-cm laceration in the right frontoparietal region, along with a depressed skull fracture and signs of acute subdural hematoma causing mass effect (**Fig. 7B.1**).

A craniotomy was performed in order to evacuate an acute subdural hematoma located in the frontal area and to elevate a depressed fracture in the temporal region. After the surgery, the patient developed notable cerebral edema

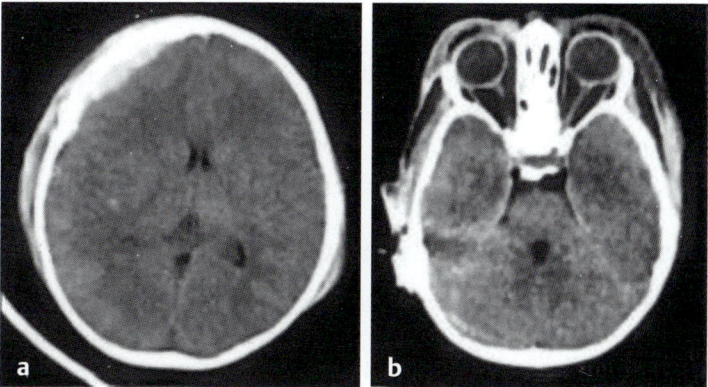

**Fig. 7B.1** **(a)** Admission axial brain CT scan showing multiple bilateral parietal fractures, right frontotemporal depressed fracture with underlying acute subdural hematoma (SDH), multiple contusions, midline shift, compression of the right lateral ventricle, effacement of sulci, and absence of cisterns. **(b)** Postoperative CT scan. Used with permission from Samer Hoz.

causing the frontoparietal lobes to shift away from the craniotomy location. Efforts to reduce brain swelling were ineffective, prompting the decision to proceed with DC, which also proved to be unsuccessful in relieving the swollen brain that impeded the closure of the scalp. Due to ventricular compression, ventricular tapping was not a feasible option, leaving cisternostomy as the sole viable alternative.

The initial step involved the subfrontal corridor being directed by the sphenoid ridge to reach the olfactory cistern, as well as the carotid, inter-optic, and chiasmatic cisterns. Following this, the cisterns were successively opened until the anterior communicating artery was identified. The opening of the cisterns led to a considerable drainage of CSF, effectively reducing brain swelling. Afterwards, the bone flap was repositioned, and the scalp closure was accomplished without any complications related to anesthesia or surgery. The surgical procedure was conducted using a surgical loupe for magnification and illumination (Zeiss ×4.3).

A postoperative CT scan showed the absence of edema, contusions, or midline shift. After the surgical procedure, the patient had a successful recovery and was discharged from the hospital in a span of 3 days. Subsequent check-ups at 6 months confirmed the patient's favorable health condition.

## Case 2: Cisternostomy in Acute Brain Swelling

A middle-aged man, aged 56, was found in an unconscious state by his spouse in the rear area of their residence, roughly half an hour subsequent to their shared evening meal. Subsequently, he was transported to the Emergency Department of the Neurosurgery Teaching Hospital situated in Baghdad, Iraq, within a 60-minute timeframe from the moment of discovery. Upon his admission, he displayed a score of 8 on the Glasgow coma scale (with individual scores of E2M4V2). Furthermore, he manifested indications of weakened functionality in the form of weakness on the left side of his body, categorized as Medical Research Council (MRC) power grade 2. Of particular note was the presence of anisocoria, wherein his right pupil measured 5 mm in diameter while the left pupil measured 3 mm, and both pupils exhibited reactivity to light stimuli.

An initial assessment was carried out. The patient's relatives gave a negative response of any past occurrences of trauma, hypertension, or diabetes mellitus, and indicated that he is dominantly right-handed. A markedly elevated blood pressure was recorded. Concurrently, a series of blood tests were conducted for rudimentary inquiries, alongside a cerebral CT scan as illustrated in **Fig. 7B.2**. The imaging displayed a substantial hemorrhage in the right putamen measuring around 60 mL, reaching depths of approximately 1 cm below the cerebral cortex, with adjacent surrounding edema leading to notable midline displacement toward the

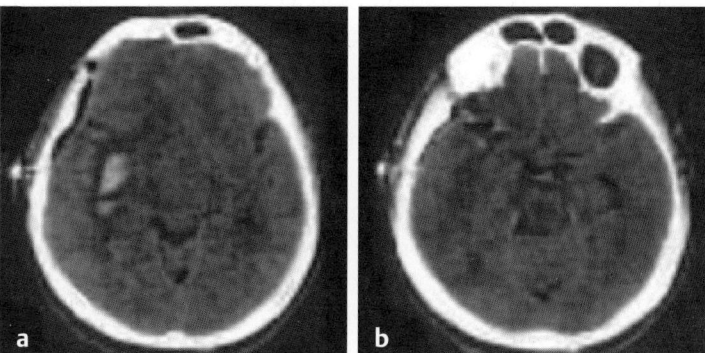

**Fig. 7B.2** An axial CT scan of the brain postoperatively reveals the following findings: **(a)** A partial removal of the hematoma with the restoration of midline shift and repositioning of the bone flap directly above a relaxed cortex. **(b)** The presence of numerous aeroceles within the basal cistern, indicative of the performed cisternostomy. Used with permission from Samer Hoz.

left and effacement of the adjacent lateral ventricle and the sulci, and the lack of basal cisterns was also observed. No signs of extension into the ventricles were detected.

The decision to perform surgery by doing a craniotomy for evacuation of hematoma was made based on a variety of factors, such as the age of the patient, rapid onset, progressing symptoms, hematoma characteristics (situated in nondominant hemisphere, significant midline shift to the left, large size, and accessibility), and absence of comorbidities. The patient's family members were extensively briefed on the indications, risks, and potential outcomes of the surgery, both with and without intervention, and their formal consent was obtained before the procedure was initiated.

The craniotomy was performed to evacuate the ICH, during which the dura mater was incised, and an incision was placed on the cerebral cortex. A partial removal of the hematoma was executed to uphold the tamponade effect over the minute, multiple bleeding foci commonly confronted in such pathological conditions. Nevertheless, as the surgical procedure advanced, there was a rapid onset of swelling of the brain, with no discernible or visible etiology noted upon examination of the hematoma location. Diverse maneuvers such as head end elevation, modifying parameters of anesthesia, assessing for any obstruction of the endotracheal tube in the form of any kink, hyperventilation, and administering a rapid IV bolus of mannitol, which all aim at brain relaxation, were employed. But in spite of these interventions, the progressive cerebral edema continued. Due to the presence of pre-existing ventricular compression detected in the preoperative CT scan, performing a ventricular tap was considered unfeasible.

To address brain herniation at the craniotomy site, we decided to perform basal cisternostomy. Using a surgical loupe (Zeiss ×4.3), a tool commonly employed in urgent situations at our institution instead of a microscope, we carried out cisternostomy on the carotid cisterns, inter-optic cisterns, and proximal sylvian cisterns. The drainage of CSF from these cisterns was maintained until the brain achieved a good state of relaxation, and this was done until we witnessed arrest of outward herniation and the reduction of swelling within the next 15-minute period. After this, we followed the standard protocol; first was securing a watertight dural closure followed by repositioning the bone flap to its original position.

The evolution of the patient's consciousness showed a notable progression in the postoperative period. The initial imaging post-surgery displayed successful removal of most of the hematoma and a correction of the midline deviation (**Fig. 7B.2**). Subsequent to this, the patient was discharged to continue recovery at home. Throughout this period, there was a persistent enhancement in the patient's awareness and a mild amelioration in the motor capability on the left side. At 1 year post the surgical procedure, the patient attained self-sufficiency with minor weakness evident in the left upper extremity. Concurrently, he had commenced employment as a cashier at a nearby restaurant.

# Proposed Classification Systems for Cisternostomy

## According to the Mechanism Involved

The ventricular system connecting to the cisternal subarachnoid space provides a pathway for the outflow or inflow system of CSF through cisternostomy. By utilizing cisternostomy, atmospheric pressure is balanced with basal cistern pressure, thereby facilitating brain relaxation to achieve its intended purpose. Therefore, the authors advocate for the classification of cisternostomy into two overarching groups as described below:

1. **Outflow passage:** A cisternostomy procedure creates a drainage outlet for CSF in the ventricles and/or enclosed fluid-filled compartments. This includes the following:

   - **Ventriculocisternostomy:** Ventriculocisternostomy is most likely to succeed when the subarachnoid spaces are open and when the floor of the third ventricle bulges into the interpeduncular cistern. The only effective treatment for obstructive hydrocephalus in cases where the underlying lesion cannot be excised is diverting ventricular CSF. The determination of the procedure is based on the extent of permeability of the subarachnoid spaces. If the subarachnoid spaces are not patent, a ventriculoatrial or ventriculoperitoneal shunt is the recommended course of action. Unfortunately, this scenario is often seen in babies and in young or adult patients with "communicating" hydrocephalus stemming from meningitis or subarachnoid hemorrhage.

   - **Ventriculocisternostomy has two primary indications:**
     - Tumoral aqueductal stenosis serves as a palliative treatment for inoperable tumors such as brain stem gliomas, or as a preparatory measure before radiotherapy or exploration of pineal region tumors.
     - On the other hand, nontumoral aqueductal stenosis in both young and adult patients presents an ideal situation for intervention.[12] The use of subfrontal endoscopic fenestration of the lamina terminalis (EFLT), interhemispheric endoscopic fenestration of the lamina terminalis (IEFLT),

and microsurgical third ventriculostomy that represents a novel approach as an alternative technique to the conventional endoscopic third ventriculostomy can be used in this concept.[13,14]

- **Cystocisternostomy:** Cystocisternostomy involves intentional fenestration and drainage in conditions such as Rathke's cleft cysts and arachnoid cysts into the subarachnoid space through cisternostomy.[15]

2. **Inflow passage (proper cisternostomy):** The concept of inflow passage states that by doing cisternostomy, we achieve bidirectional pathway and it allows exit of CSF in order to relax brain during the procedures done for ruptured aneurysm, arteriovenous malformation (AVM), tumors, and ICH and in severe TBI it allows egress of blood into subarachnoid space, thus aiming to equalize the intraparenchymal pressure with intracisternal pressure.[1]

The inflow cisternostomy can be divided into convexity and basal cisternostomy. The basal cisternostomy is further categorized into supratentorial and infratentorial. Among these, the proper cisternostomy procedure is the basal supratentorial cisternostomy[16] (**Flowchart 7B.1**).

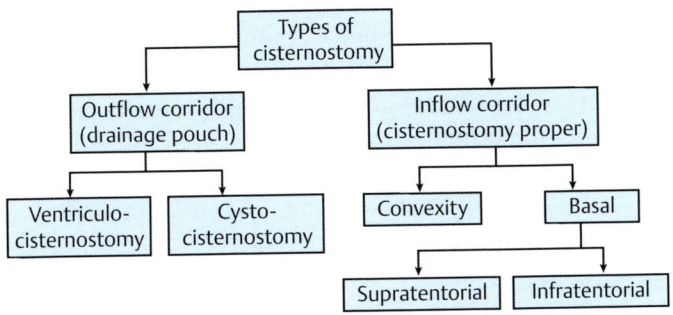

**Flowchart 7B.1** Classification of cisternostomy based on the mechanism. Used with permission from Samer Hoz.

## Classification of Cisternostomy Proper According to the Indications

The technical procedure in which we open the basal cistern of the supratentorial region into the subarachnoid space which is present infratentorially by creating fenestrations of specific cisterns such as the opticocarotid, proximal sylvian, chiasmatic, and suprasellar cisterns along with fenestration of Liliequist membrane is defined as cisternostomy, and this was outlined by Cherian et al.[16] On reviewing various literatures on the different indications for cisternostomy, these indications led to the emergence of two groups, namely, planned and unplanned cisternostomy.

Planned cisternostomy encompasses the uncomplicated or simple cisternostomy employed in procedures involving the skull base for the treatment of tumors, along with microsurgical techniques for aneurysms, AVMs, and ICH. Moreover, it can be implemented within the framework of the emerging concept of CSF shift-induced edema, thereby positioning cisternostomy as a viable alternative to DC.

The unplanned cisternostomy is done at instances of intraoperative cerebral swelling during craniotomy for brain pathology. In these cases, cisternostomy can invert the direction of CSF displacement, resulting in decreased brain swelling. Moreover, this method can mitigate pressure within the paravascular regions and interstitium, thereby promoting the restoration of paravascular system functionality[17] (**Flowchart 7B.2**).

## Conclusion

Given its demonstrated efficacy and benefits as exemplified in the preceding cases, particularly in situations considered challenging neurosurgical cases, cisternostomy emerges as

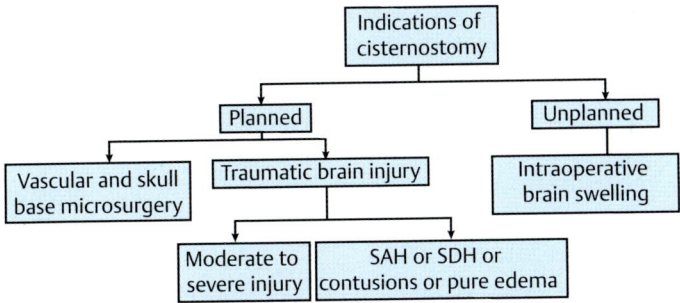

**Flowchart 7B.2** Classification of cisternostomy proper based on the indications. Used with permission from Samer Hoz.

a novel surgical technique warranting dissemination and global adoption among neurosurgeons worldwide, owing to the specialized training it necessitates.

## Suggested Readings

Carney N, Totten AM, O'Reilly C, et al. Guidelines for the Management of Severe Traumatic Brain Injury, Fourth Edition. Neurosurgery 2017;80(1):6–15

Hoz SS, Alramadan AH, Hadi AQ, Moscote Salazar LR. Cisternostomy in neurosurgery: a new proposed general classification based on mechanism and indications of the cisternostomy proper. J Neurosci Rural Pract 2018;9(4):650–652

Hutchinson PJ, Kolias AG, Timofeev IS, et al; RESCUEicp Trial Collaborators. Trial of decompressive craniectomy for traumatic intracranial hypertension. N Engl J Med 2016;375(12): 1119–1130

## References

1. Cherian I, Bernardo A, Grasso G. Cisternostomy for traumatic brain injury: pathophysiologic mechanisms and surgical technical notes. World Neurosurg 2016;89:51–57

2. Grasso G. Surgical treatment for traumatic brain injury: is it time for reappraisal? World Neurosurg 2015;84(2):594

3. Masoudi MS, Rezaee E, Hakiminejad H, Tavakoli M, Sadeghpoor T. Cisternostomy for management of intracranial hypertension in severe traumatic brain injury; case report and literature review. Bull Emerg Trauma 2016;4(3):161–164

4. Abdulqader MN, Al-Tameemi AH, Salih H, Hoz SS, Al Ramadan AH, Salazar LR. Acute intra-operative brain swelling managed effectively with emergency basal cisternostomy: a case report. J Acute Dis 2018;7(1):43–44

5. Ganau M, Prisco L. Comment on "neuromonitoring in traumatic brain injury." Minerva Anestesiol 2013;79(3):310–311

6. Zahraa A, Al-Sharshahi F. Basal cisternostomy proper for acute external brain herniation during craniotomy: a case report.

7. Yang L, Kress BT, Weber HJ, et al. Evaluating glymphatic pathway function utilizing clinically relevant intrathecal infusion of CSF tracer. J Transl Med 2013;11:107

8. Iliff JJ, Wang M, Liao Y, et al. A paravascular pathway facilitates CSF flow through the brain parenchyma and the clearance of interstitial solutes, including amyloid β. Sci Transl Med 2012;4(147):147ra111

9. Kanmounye US. The rise of inflow cisternostomy in resource-limited settings: rationale, limitations, and future challenges. Emerg Med Int 2021;2021:6630050

10. Gnanakumar S, Abou El Ela Bourqiun B, Robertson FC. The World Federation of Neurosurgical Societies Young Neurosurgeons Survey (Part I): demographics, resources, and education. World Neurosurg X 2020;8:100083

11. Dewan MC, Baticulon RE, Rattani A, Johnston JM, Warf BC, Harkness W. Pediatric neurosurgical workforce, access to care, equipment and training needs worldwide. Neurosurg Focus 2018;45(4):E13

12. Guiot G. Ventriculo-cisternostomy for stenosis of the aqueduct of Sylvius. Puncture of the floor of the third ventricle with a leucotome under television control. Acta Neurochir (Wien) 1973;28(4):275–289

13. van Lindert EJ. Microsurgical third ventriculocisternostomy as an alternative to ETV: report of two cases. Childs Nerv Syst 2008;24(6):757–761

14. Beer-Furlan A, Pinto FG, Evins AI, et al. Interhemispheric endoscopic fenestration of the lamina terminalis through a single frontal burr hole. J Neurol Surg B Skull Base 2014;75(4):268–272

15. Su Y, Ishii Y, Lin CM, Tahara S, Teramoto A, Morita A. Endoscopic transsphenoidal cisternostomy for nonneoplastic sellar cysts. BioMed Res Int 2015;2015:389474

16. Cherian I, Grasso G, Bernardo A, Munakomi S. Anatomy and physiology of cisternostomy. Chin J Traumatol 2016;19(1):7–10

17. Cherian I, Beltran M, Landi A, Alafaci C, Torregrossa F, Grasso G. Introducing the concept of "CSF-shift edema" in traumatic brain injury. J Neurosci Res 2018;96(4):744–752

# 7C Perspective about Basal Cisternostomy

*Manish Jaiswal and Sarita Kumari*

## Introduction

Traumatic brain injury leads to substantial morbidity and mortality. Development of intracranial hypertension in the setting of traumatic brain injury results in poorer prognosis and is a key factor for development of secondary brain injury. Management of traumatic brain injury mainly focus on minimizing or controlling this secondary brain injury.

Decompressive craniectomy procedure has proven its role in decreasing intracranial pressure and mortality. Whether this translates into favorable or unfavorable outcome is still under debate. Moreover, decompressive craniectomy procedure has its own set of complications that include external cerebral herniation, blooming of contusions, subdural/ epidural hematoma contralateral to craniectomy defect, strangulation of cerebral tissue at edge of bone flap that can lead to infarction, delayed postoperative seizures, neurological deterioration and subdural hygromas, hydrocephalus, and syndrome of trephine at later stage.

The pathophysiological basis for these complications is based on the fact that decompressive craniectomy helps in reducing intracranial pressure but not intracerebral pressure. It provides an outlet for edematous brain to expand manifesting as vegetative state or severe disabilities later.

This leads to alterations in compliance, cerebral blood flow, autoregulation and cerebrospinal fluid (CSF) circulation, and disruption of the subarachnoid CSF pathways. To address this issue, basal cisternostomy has been recently proposed as an alternative or adjunctive technique which has the potential to reduce intracranial pressure as well as brain edema.

As opposed to previous concepts of CSF circulation, the new concept states that CSF is continuously produced, absorbed, and circulated in the entire CSF system. Paravascular Virchow-Robin spaces forming glymphatic system plays a major role in that. In traumatic brain injury, this glymphatic system gets impaired because of traumatic subarachnoid hemorrhage (SAH) that clogs natural CSF pathways leading to decrease in interstitial fluid drainage and hence brain edema. By opening basal cisterns and lamina terminalis, cisternal pressure is decreased reversing shift of fluid from intraparenchymal to cisternal compartment, thus alleviating brain swelling.

## Our Perspective

- Our experience concluded that basal cisternostomy is an effective procedure in reducing both intracranial pressure as well as brain edema. While performing basal cisternostomy, basal cisterns like (peri-chiasmatic cisterns, carotid cisterns, suprasellar cisterns, and interpeduncular cistern) are opened along with fenestration of Liliequist membrane. This leads to release of CSF and allows extensive washout and clearing of blood clots/debris from cisternal spaces. In response, glymphatic pathway and normal CSF circulation pathways become functional again. This results in reduction in both intracranial pressure as well as brain edema, hence decreasing the risk of secondary brain injury. The minimization of secondary brain injury translates into clinically relevant improvement in patient outcome like shorter duration of ventilatory support and ICU stay, better Glasgow coma scale (GCS) and Glasgow Outcome Scale–Extended (GOS-E) scores, and lesser tendency of seizure development in the postoperative period.

- In cases where basal cisterns are open in preoperative scan, release of CSF leads to immediate relaxation of brain and replacement of bone flap at craniotomy site during primary surgery was possible. The authors also noticed that in cases where basal cisterns are obliterated in preoperative scan, no CSF release is seen on opening cisterns so brain laxity achieved in these cases is not adequate for making bone flap replacement possible. However, clinical improvement is seen in these cases due to cleaning and opening of clogged cisternal spaces that make glymphatic and CSF circulatory pathways functional again, therefore reducing brain edema and secondary brain injury.

- In cases where bone flap placement is possible, need for second surgery for cranioplasty is obviated. As a result, complications associated with decompressive craniectomy or second surgery can be avoided. In cases where bone flap could not be replaced during primary surgery early cranioplasty is possible.

Due to re-establishment of normal circulatory pathways and CSF dynamics, there is lesser risk of post-traumatic hydrocephalus in patients who undergo basal cisternostomy procedure.

## Limitations

In spite of being a promising procedure, its application is not widespread.

Following limitations hinders its practice in trauma cases which are generally taken care of by residents:

- Requirement of microscope in trauma setup.
- Mandate for a surgeon skilled in skull base and micro-neurosurgery.

Reaching up to and opening basal cisterns is a herculean task in unskilled hands and trickier in an edematous brain even in skilled hands. To combat this issue adequate training should be provided to younger generation. There are certain technical points that can be incorporated to make it feasible:

- Patient's head positioning is one of the key factors for a safe trajectory to cisterns. This also minimizes the need for static retraction.
- Evacuation of hematoma and contusion can be done first in cases where brain is bulging. It makes approaching basal cisterns less cumbersome.

Some surgeons prefer anterior clinoid process drilling for approaching basal cisterns. Some difficult cases required posterior clinoid process drilling as well for proper visualization. Drilling of anterior clinoid process in edematous brain has added risk of injuring internal carotid artery in unexperienced hands. The authors were able to reach the cisterns with sphenoid ridge drilling and using lateral subfrontal approach, and they do not advice drilling of clinoid process for proper visualization.

After opening dura, brain spatula can be used to retract the brain. Use of static retraction with brain spatula in a traumatized edematous brain might lead to further injury.

Hence, use of dynamic retraction with working instruments is advised in place of static retraction to avoid or minimize injury to brain.

## Conclusion

With proper training, younger generation can be trained effortlessly so that the benefits of this procedure, if any, can be extended to a wider population.

As cisternostomy procedure offers multitude of benefits, therefore in the authors' opinion basal cisternostomy should be performed in all cases if required skill and resources are available.

# 7D Perspectives on Cisternostomy and Case Scenarios

*Ramesh Chandra*

## Introduction

The glymphatic system demonstrates that cerebrospinal fluid (CSF) from the cisterns communicates with the brain parenchyma through the Virchow-Robin spaces (VRS). A recognized method for reducing intracranial pressure (ICP) involves evacuating CSF by opening the basal subarachnoid cisterns. Traumatic brain injury (TBI) is a significant cause of morbidity and mortality worldwide. It consists of primary and secondary brain injuries, with the latter resulting from brain swelling and increased ICP. Although decompressive hemicraniectomy has been the standard surgical approach for managing TBI, it has its own complications. Cisternostomy, a novel surgical technique, entails opening the basal subarachnoid cisterns to reduce ICP by utilizing the CSF communication pathways between the brain parenchyma (Virchow-Robin spaces) and the cisternal spaces.

Cisternostomy is indicated in moderate to severe head injury and the indications include, but are not restricted to, drop in Glasgow Coma Scale (GCS) motor score with signs of ipsilateral cerebellopontine angle (CPA) cistern widening in unilateral acute subdural hematoma (SDH) causing mass effect, subarachnoid hemorrhage with brain swelling, unilateral single contusion with mild to moderate mass effect (with or without SDH), unilateral multiple contusions with brain swelling (also with or without SDH), and bilateral contusions along with bilateral subdural hematomas resulting in brain swelling.

A scoring system was developed to help in guiding the clinician to decide about cisternostomy. The scoring termed as cisternostomy indication score takes into consideration three parameters **(Table 7D.1)** and management is based on the total score **(Table 7D.2)**.

**Table 7D.1**   Cisternostomy indication score on the basis of MPC

| GCS motor score | (M) | Pupil status | (P) | Cisterns on computed tomography | (C) |
|---|---|---|---|---|---|
| M2/M1 | 0 | Bilaterally dilated and nonreactive | 0 | Complete herniation with brain stem torsion and/or PCA infarction | 0 |
| M3 | 1 | Unilaterally dilated and nonreactive | 1 | Cerebellopontine angle obliterated | 1 |
| M4 | 2 | Unilaterally dilated and reactive | 2 | Suprasellar cisterns obliterated and CPA cistern widened | 2 |
| M5 | 3 | Normal | 3 | All cisterns open | 3 |
| M6 | 4 | | | | |
| **TOTAL SCORE (M + P + C).** | | | | | |

Abbreviations: CPA: cerebellopontine angle; GCS: Glasgow Coma Scale; PCA: Posterior cerebral artery.

**Table 7D.2**   Management on the basis of the total CIS

| Total CIS score | Management |
|---|---|
| 9–10 | Conservative treatment and close neurological follow-up recommended |
| 8 | Depending on the clinical progression and the clinical scenario, either a close watch or cisternostomy |
| 3–7 | Cisternostomy is indicated if no diffuse axonal injury seen |
| 0–2 | Cisternostomy is not useful |

**Performing cisternostomy in patients with a CIS of 8 or 0–2 is subject to clinical assessment.**

Abbreviation: CIS, Cisternostomy Indication Scores.

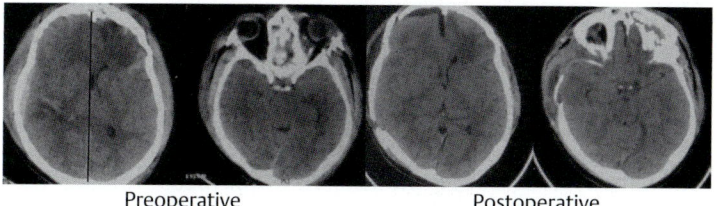
Preoperative                                    Postoperative

**Fig. 7D.1**   Preoperative and postoperative CT of a patient following frontotemporal craniotomy and basal cisternostomy.

## Case Scenarios

### Case 1

A 35-year-old male presented with a history of head injury following a fall from a two-wheeler. His GCS score was 7 out of 15 (E1V1M5). Pupils were asymmetric, with the right pupil measuring 3 mm and the left pupil measuring 3.5 mm, both reacting to light. A computed tomography (CT) scan of the brain revealed an acute SDH on the right side, causing mass effect (**Fig. 7D.1**). The total cisternostomy indication score was 6. The patient underwent a right frontotemporal craniotomy for evacuation of the SDH, along with basal cisternostomy.

## Case 2

A 39-year-old male presented with a history of head injury following a fall from a two-wheeler. His GCS score was 9 out of 15 (E2V2M5). Pupils were asymmetric, with the right pupil measuring 3.5 mm and the left pupil measuring 3 mm, both reacting to light. A CT scan of the brain revealed a right temporal contusion and an acute SDH with mass effect (**Fig. 7D.2**). The total cisternostomy indication score was 7. The patient underwent a right frontotemporal craniotomy for evacuation of the contusion and acute SDH, along with cisternostomy.

## Case 3

A 40-year-old male presented with a history of head injury following a fall from a two-wheeler. His GCS score was 8 out of 15 (E2V1M5). Pupils were asymmetric, with the right pupil measuring 3 mm and the left pupil measuring 3.5 mm, both reacting to light. A CT scan of the brain revealed a left temporal contusion with mass effect (**Fig. 7D.3**). The total cisternostomy indication score was 6. The patient underwent

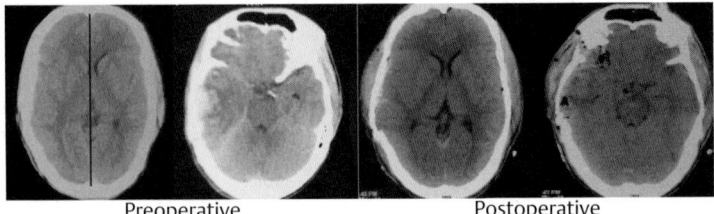

Preoperative                    Postoperative

**Fig. 7D.2** Preoperative and postoperative CT of a patient with total cisternostomy indication score of 7.

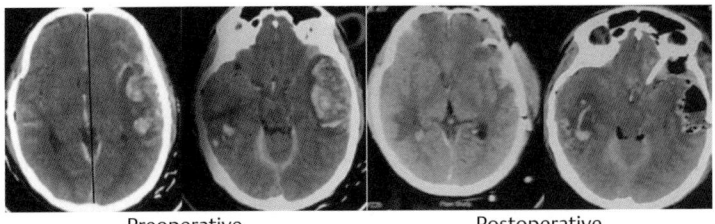

Preoperative                    Postoperative

**Fig. 7D.3**  Preoperative and postoperative CT of a patient following left frontotemporal craniotomy and basal cisternostomy.

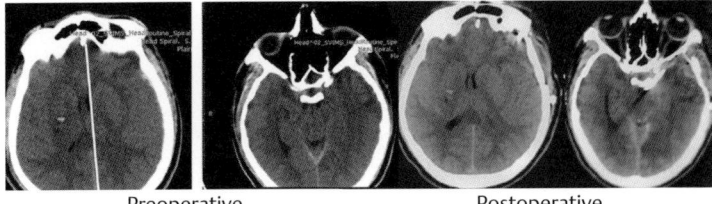

Preoperative                    Postoperative

**Fig. 7D.4**  Preoperative and postoperative CT of a patient following frontotemporal craniotomy and basal cisternostomy.

a left frontotemporal craniotomy for evacuation of the contusion, along with cisternostomy.

## Case 4

A 24-year-old male presented with a history of head injury following a fall from height. His GCS score was 7 out of 15 (E2VTM5). Pupils were asymmetric, with the right pupil measuring 3 mm and the left pupil measuring 3.5 mm, both reacting to light. A CT scan of the brain revealed a left thin acute SDH with diffuse cerebral edema **(Fig. 7D.4)**. The ICP recording was high. The total cisternostomy indication score was 8. The patient underwent a left frontotemporal craniotomy for evacuation of the SDH, along with cisternostomy.

## Conclusion

Cisternostomy, when performed judiciously, can yield outcomes comparable to decompressive craniotomy while avoiding the need for a second procedure. The key lies in careful case selection to prevent complications and maintain the procedure's reputation. Beginners can benefit from using the Total Cisternostomy Indication Scores (CIS) as a guide for case selection.

# Cisternostomy in Traumatic Brain Injury: A Breakthrough for Low- and Middle-Income Countries

**8**

*Manuel de Jesus Encarnacion Ramirez, Ismael Antonio, Peralta Baez, and Carlos Salvador Ovalle Torres*

## Introduction

Traumatic brain injury (TBI) is a significant cause of morbidity and mortality worldwide, with a disproportionately high burden in low- and middle-income countries (LMICs). The global incidence of TBI is estimated to be 69 million people annually, with the majority of cases occurring in LMICs due to factors such as road traffic accidents, falls, and violence. In these regions, limited healthcare resources and infrastructure exacerbate the challenges of managing TBI, necessitating cost-effective and efficacious interventions.

Cisternostomy is a neurosurgical procedure aimed at managing intracranial hypertension (ICH), a common and dangerous consequence of severe TBI. Traditional methods for controlling ICH, such as decompressive craniectomy (DC), have been associated with significant complications and suboptimal outcomes. Cisternostomy offers a novel approach by directly targeting the subarachnoid cisterns, which are natural cerebrospinal fluid (CSF) reservoirs located at the base of the brain. The primary objective of cisternostomy is to restore the brain's natural CSF dynamics and reduce intracranial pressure (ICP) by creating an alternative pathway for CSF drainage.

## Advantages of Cisternostomy in TBI Management

Cisternostomy presents several advantages over traditional TBI management techniques, making it particularly suitable for LMICs:

- **Reduced complications:** Compared to DC, cisternostomy is associated with lower rates of infection, bone flap resorption, and other complications. This is crucial in settings where postoperative care and infection control are challenging.
- **Improved outcomes**: Studies have shown that cisternostomy can significantly reduce ICP and improve neurological outcomes. Patients undergoing cisternostomy often exhibit better recovery trajectories and reduced long-term disability.
- **Cost-effectiveness:** Cisternostomy, being a less invasive procedure with fewer complications, can reduce overall healthcare costs. This is particularly important in LMICs where financial resources are limited.
- **Feasibility and scalability:** The procedure can be performed with standard neurosurgical instruments

and does not require advanced technological infrastructure, making it feasible for implementation in resource-limited settings.

# Limitations of Cisternostomy

Despite its potential benefits, cisternostomy has several limitations that need to be addressed to maximize its efficacy and safety in the management of TBI, particularly in LMICs.

## Technical Complexity

- **Surgical expertise:** Cisternostomy requires precise surgical skills and a thorough understanding of neuroanatomy. The complexity of the procedure can be a significant barrier, especially in LMICs where neurosurgical expertise may be limited.
- **Training and expertise:** Neurosurgeons must undergo specialized training to master cisternostomy. In LMICs, where opportunities for advanced neurosurgical training may be scarce, this poses a considerable challenge. Training programs must be developed and implemented to ensure surgeons acquire the necessary skills.
- **Learning curve**: Like many advanced surgical procedures, cisternostomy has a steep learning curve. Surgeons new to the technique may require substantial practice and supervision to achieve proficiency, increasing the risk of complications during the initial phase of adoption.

## Technological Considerations

- **Basic surgical instruments:** Cisternostomy can be performed with standard neurosurgical tools, which makes it accessible compared to more technologically demanding procedures.

- **Operative microscope:** An operative microscope provides enhanced visualization of intricate brain structures, allowing neurosurgeons to perform delicate procedures like cisternostomy with greater precision and safety. The microscope magnifies the surgical field, improving the ability to navigate around critical brain structures and reducing the risk of intraoperative complications.

## Challenges in Latin America

- **Limited availability:** In many parts of Latin America, access to operative microscopes is limited due to financial constraints and inadequate healthcare infrastructure. These microscopes are expensive, and the cost of maintenance and repair further adds to the financial burden, making them unaffordable for many healthcare facilities.

- **Resource allocation:** Healthcare budgets in LMICs, including many Latin American countries, are often stretched thin, prioritizing basic healthcare needs over specialized equipment like operative microscopes. This lack of investment hampers the ability to perform cisternostomy safely and effectively.

- **Limited evidence base**: Although emerging data is promising, the evidence base for cisternostomy is still developing. Large-scale randomized controlled trials are needed to definitively establish its efficacy and safety.

- **Postoperative care needs:** Effective postoperative monitoring and care are essential for successful outcomes. In LMICs, where intensive care units (ICUs) and neurocritical care expertise may be limited, this presents a significant challenge.

## Addressing the Limitations

To overcome these challenges and successfully integrate cisternostomy into TBI management protocols in LMICs, a multifaceted approach is required:

- Investment in equipment: There needs to be increased investment in acquiring operative microscopes for healthcare facilities across Latin America. Governments, nongovernmental organizations (NGOs), and international health agencies can play a crucial role in funding and facilitating the procurement of these essential tools.
- Training programs: Establishing training programs focused on the use of operative microscopes is essential. These programs can be facilitated through international collaborations, workshops, and telemedicine platforms, enabling neurosurgeons in Latin America to gain the necessary skills to use the microscopes effectively.
- Telemedicine and remote support: Leveraging telemedicine for remote consultation and support can help bridge the gap in expertise. Experienced neurosurgeons from around the world can provide real-time guidance and support to their counterparts in Latin America during cisternostomy procedures, ensuring the safe and effective use of operative microscopes.
- Public–private partnerships: Forming public–private partnerships can help secure funding for the acquisition and maintenance of operative microscopes. Collaborations with medical device manufacturers can also facilitate access to affordable equipment and training.

# Regional Applications and Case Studies

## Mexico

In Mexico, the integration of cisternostomy into TBI management protocols has shown promising results. Several neurosurgical centers have adopted the procedure, driven by the need to improve outcomes for TBI patients. Collaborative efforts between local neurosurgeons and international experts have facilitated training and capacity building. Early outcomes indicate that cisternostomy can significantly reduce ICP and improve neurological recovery, making it a valuable addition to the neurosurgical repertoire in Mexico.

## Dominican Republic

Dr. Ismael Peralta and Manuel Encarnacion Ramirez have been pioneering figures in introducing cisternostomy in the Dominican Republic. Their research and clinical practice have demonstrated the procedure's potential to transform TBI care in the region. Their first research highlight the importance of tailored training programs and the need for a multidisciplinary approach to optimize outcomes. Their work underscores the feasibility of cisternostomy in settings with limited resources, advocating for its broader adoption across the Caribbean region.

## Russia

In the Russia Federation, Manuel Encarnacion Ramirez published the first series of cases of cisternostomy. Cisternostomy has been a part of ongoing efforts to enhance TBI care. Russian neurosurgeons have reported success in using cisternostomy to manage severe TBI, with a focus on reducing secondary brain injury and improving functional outcomes. The experience in Russia highlights the importance of integrating new surgical techniques with existing protocols and emphasizes the need for continuous research and innovation.

# Strategies for Implementation in LMICs

To successfully integrate cisternostomy into TBI management protocols in LMICs, a comprehensive and multifaceted strategy is essential. This strategy must address training, infrastructure, community engagement, research, and policy advocacy to overcome the unique challenges faced by these regions.

## Capacity Building

Neurosurgical training programs:

- International collaborations: Establish partnerships with established neurosurgical centers and academic institutions globally to facilitate knowledge transfer. This can include exchange programs, fellowships, and visiting scholar initiatives where LMIC neurosurgeons can receive hands-on training in advanced centers.
- Workshops and conferences: Regularly organize workshops, conferences, and seminars focused on cisternostomy techniques. These events can be held in LMICs and led by international experts, providing practical training and theoretical knowledge.
- Telemedicine and e-learning platforms: Utilize telemedicine for real-time consultations and e-learning platforms to provide continuous education. Virtual training modules, webinars, and online courses can help neurosurgeons in LMICs stay updated with the latest advancements and best practices in cisternostomy.

## Development of Local Expertise

- Mentorship programs: Implement mentorship programs where experienced neurosurgeons guide and support less experienced colleagues through the learning curve of cisternostomy.
- Simulation training: Establish simulation centers equipped with advanced models and virtual reality systems to provide risk-free environments for practicing cisternostomy procedures.

## Resource Allocation

Investment in infrastructure:

- Government and NGO support: Advocate for increased funding from governments, NGOs, and international health agencies to improve neurosurgical infrastructure. This includes upgrading operating rooms, ensuring a steady supply of essential surgical instruments, and maintaining sterile environments.
- Public–private partnerships: Foster collaborations between the public sector and private companies to fund the acquisition and maintenance of operative microscopes and other critical equipment. Medical device manufacturers can offer subsidized rates or donations to support healthcare facilities in LMICs.
- Ensuring availability of critical equipment
- Operative microscopes or exoscopes: Secure the provision of operative microscopes or exoscopes, which are essential for the precision required in cisternostomy. Implement regular maintenance schedules and establish local partnerships for equipment repair and servicing.

- Preoperative imaging: Improve access to advanced imaging modalities such as CT and MRI scanners. This can be achieved through investments in portable imaging technology and mobile units that can serve multiple facilities.

## Community Engagement

Educational campaigns:

- Healthcare providers: Conduct targeted educational campaigns to inform healthcare providers about the benefits and protocols of cisternostomy. This includes workshops for emergency room doctors, nurses, and paramedics to recognize TBI symptoms and refer patients promptly.
- Public awareness: Launch public awareness campaigns to educate communities about TBI prevention, early symptoms, and the potential benefits of cisternostomy. Utilize various media platforms, including radio, television, and social media, to reach a broad audience.

## Addressing Cultural and Socioeconomic Barriers

- Community involvement: Engage community leaders and local organizations to support the dissemination of information and foster trust in the healthcare system. Addressing cultural beliefs and misconceptions about brain surgery can enhance acceptance and cooperation.
- Financial support programs: Develop financial assistance programs for patients and families to alleviate the economic burden of surgery and postoperative care. Collaborate with local charities and international aid organizations to provide funding and resources.

## Research and Data Collection

Establishing registries:

- National and regional databases: Create national and regional TBI registries to systematically collect data on patient outcomes, complications, and long-term recovery following cisternostomy. This data is crucial for monitoring the procedure's effectiveness and identifying areas for improvement.
- Collaborative research networks: Form collaborative research networks involving multiple healthcare institutions in LMICs. This will facilitate large-scale studies and enable data sharing, contributing to a more robust evidence base for cisternostomy.

## Conducting Clinical Trials

- Randomized controlled trials (RCTs): Initiate and support RCTs to compare cisternostomy with traditional TBI management techniques. These trials should focus on patient outcomes, cost-effectiveness, and the feasibility of implementation in resource-limited settings.
- Post-implementation studies: Conduct post-implementation studies to assess the long-term impact of cisternostomy on patient outcomes and healthcare systems. These studies can help refine protocols and demonstrate the procedure's sustainability and scalability.

## Policy Advocacy

Integration into national guidelines:

- Policy development: Advocate for the inclusion of cisternostomy in national TBI management guidelines. This involves engaging with policymakers, healthcare authorities, and professional societies to highlight the procedure's benefits and evidence base.

- Standardized protocols: Develop and disseminate standardized protocols for cisternostomy, ensuring consistency in its application across various healthcare facilities. These protocols should be tailored to the specific needs and constraints of LMICs.

## Conclusion

Traumatic brain injuries were dealt with a primitive surgical option, i.e., decompressive hemicraniectomy, for last 50 years. Cisternostomy is a paradigm shift with microneurosurgical principles being used in trauma. Although the results are much better, the procedure of cisternostomy needs a complete change in mindset, infrastructure, and skill, which is difficult in the third world countries without much infrastructure back-up. However, considering the trauma load in these countries, a paradigm shift in infrastructure mindset and training needs to be undertaken for the best results in trauma.

## Suggested Readings

Allen BC, Cummer E, Sarma AK. Traumatic brain injury in select low- and middle-income countries: a narrative review of the literature. J Neurotrauma 2023;40(7-8):602–619

De Jesus Encarnacion Ramirez M, Peralta I, Ramirez I, et al. Development of a novel low-cost exoscope to expand access to microneurosurgical care in low- and middle-income countries. World Neurosurg 2022;163:5–10

Encarnación Ramirez M, Baez IP, Mukengeshay JN, et al. The role of cisternostomy in the management of severe traumatic brain injury: a triple-center study. Surgeries (Basel) 2023;4(2): 283–292

Encarnacion Ramirez MJ, Barrientos Castillo RE, Vorobiev A, Kiselev N, Aquino AA, Efe IE. Basal cisternostomy for traumatic brain injury: a case report of unexpected good recovery. Chin J Traumatol 2022;25(5):302–305

Kumar P, Goyal N, Chaturvedi J, et al. Basal cisternostomy in head injury: more questions than answers. Neurol India 2022;70(4): 1384–1390

Rivera-Lara L, Videtta W, Calvillo E, et al. Reducing the incidence and mortality of traumatic brain injury in Latin America. Eur J Trauma Emerg Surg 2023;49(6):2381–2388

Samanamalee S, Sigera PC, De Silva AP, et al. Traumatic brain injury (TBI) outcomes in an LMIC tertiary care centre and performance of trauma scores. BMC Anesthesiol 2018;18(1):4

Shakir M, Altaf A, Irshad HA, et al. Factors delaying the continuum of care for the management of traumatic brain injury in lowand middle-income countries: a systematic review. World Neurosurg 2023;180:169–193.e3

Volovici V, Haitsma IK. Cisternostomy in traumatic brain injury: time for the world to listen—cerebrospinal fluid release: possibly the missing link in traumatic brain injury. World Neurosurg 2022;162:3–5

# Review of Literature on Cisternostomy

**9**

*Kodeeswaran M., Priyadharshan K. P., Chirag Hiran, and Naveen Kumar M.*

## Introduction

Brain edema following severe traumatic brain injury (TBI) is a critical factor influencing patient outcomes and survival. It is a key focus in current clinical treatment strategies. The pathophysiology of traumatic brain swelling, which includes cytotoxic and vasogenic origins, remains complex and not fully elucidated. Recent insights into the hydrodynamic properties of cerebrospinal fluid (CSF) suggest an additional mechanism of brain swelling known as "CSF-shift edema." This mechanism involves increased pressure in the subarachnoid space, leading to a rapid shift of CSF into the brain through paravascular spaces, resulting in increased brain water content. The CSF shift, driven by a pressure gradient, elevates pressure within paravascular spaces and brain interstitium, disrupting paravascular system functions and potentially causing secondary brain injury. Cisternostomy, an innovative surgical intervention, can reverse the CSF shift, reducing brain swelling by altering the direction of CSF flow. This procedure can alleviate pressure in paravascular spaces and interstitium, restoring paravascular system functionality and aiding recovery. Cisternostomy presents a promising solution by redirecting CSF flow to restore optimal pressure levels in the brain, offering a novel approach to managing brain swelling. A novel approach to addressing brain swelling involves utilizing cisternostomy to redirect CSF flow and restore normal pressure levels within the brain.[1]

In the year 2013, a study was done by Iype Cherian et al in the College of Medical Sciences, Hebei University[2] which applied the principles of microvascular surgery and skull base surgery in select cases of severe traumatic brain injuries, thereby replacing decompressive hemicraniectomy as the primary modality of treatment for indicated cases. This innovative approach aims to address brain edema following severe TBI by leveraging microvascular and skull base surgical techniques to manage brain swelling more effectively. By implementing these specialized surgical strategies, the study aimed to improve patient outcomes and survival rates in cases of severe TBI.

In the year 2016, Mohammad Sadegh Masoudi and others reported a case involving a 13-year-old boy who suffered severe TBI following a motor vehicle accident and demonstrated the successful use of cisternostomy as a treatment approach.[3] This alternative technique proved effective in controlling intracranial pressure (ICP) and managing refractory intracranial hypertension in the patient. The boy presented with diffuse brain edema, a left frontal contusion, and a posterior interhemispheric subdural hematoma, with ICP monitoring indicating a mean value of 26 mmHg. The decision to perform cisternostomy led to a significant improvement in the patient's neurological status within hours post-surgery. Subsequent recovery progress was notable, with the boy being discharged from the hospital after 5 days and achieving complete recovery during the 3-month follow-up period. This case underscores the potential of cisternostomy as a successful alternative to decompressive craniectomy (DC) in managing severe TBI cases with intracranial hypertension.

DC is widely acknowledged as the primary surgical intervention for refractory cerebral edema in cases of TBI. Its primary benefit lies in the reduction of intracranial pressure (ICP) through the creation of space for the swollen brain tissue. Efforts are currently underway to explore alternative procedures that could potentially enhance outcomes in TBI cases. One such approach, basal cisternostomy, has been proposed and discussed in the existing body of literature. An investigation conducted by Jutty K. B. C. Parthiban et al5 aimed to evaluate the efficacy of basal cisternostomy in patients with TBI. The retrospective analysis involved a cohort of 40 TBI patients who underwent basal cisternostomy while under treatment in the senior author's facility between January 2016 and April 2019. All surgical interventions were carried out by a single surgeon with specialized expertise in microsurgery. The assessment of outcomes was based on the GOS, and statistical analysis was performed using SPSS software. The findings indicated that in cases of severe TBI, the basal cisternostomy group exhibited a favorable outcome of 77.8%, compared to 72.7% in the group that underwent DC alongside basal bisternostomy. Of the total cohort, 82% (33/40) experienced a favorable GOS outcome, while 12.5% (5/40) had an unfavorable outcome, and 5% (2/40) resulted in mortality. Incidences of hydrocephalus were observed in 12.5% (5/40) of cases. Patients who underwent surgery promptly following the injury demonstrated superior outcomes compared to those who had delayed procedures, regardless of the initial neurological status. Unfortunately, the assessment of ICU and hospital stay durations could not be conclusive.

But in the year 2020, Omar Youssef et al4 held the opinion that surgical removal of acute subdural hematoma (ASDH) has remained the primary treatment approach for patients with ASDH who exhibit progressive neurological deficits, escalating ICP, or significant mass effect. Cisternostomy involves the opening of the basal cisterns with the aim of equalizing their pressure with atmospheric conditions, thereby reducing the intraparenchymal pressure. The objective of this study was to assess the impact of incorporating cisternostomy into decompressive craniotomy on the outcomes of patients with traumatic ASDH. A total of 40 patients meeting specific criteria were included in the study, presenting at Cairo University hospital emergency department between January 2018 and June 2019. The inclusion criteria encompassed an age range of 12 to 65 years, traumatic ASDH with a thickness of ≥10 mm or midline shift of ≥5 mm, and a Glasgow coma scale (GCS) score upon admission of <10, without accompanying intraparenchymal hematoma of ≥1 cm or severe comorbidities. The patients were randomly assigned to two groups based on their arrival sequence. The first group underwent decompressive craniotomy (DHC) along with cisternostomy, while the second group received decompressive craniotomy alone. Evaluation of outcomes was conducted using the Glasgow outcome score (GOS). The results indicated a relatively better outcome in the first group (DHC + cisternostomy) compared to the second group (DHC only), although the differences were not statistically significant. Mortality rates were 35% (7/20 patients) in the first group and 50% (10/20 patients) in the second group, with median GOS of 3 and 1, respectively. The addition of cisternostomy to decompressive craniotomy led to a mean increase in surgical duration of 35.5 minutes. Advanced age and lower GCS upon admission were associated with notably poorer outcomes in our analysis. In conclusion, the study findings suggest that supplementing decompressive craniotomy with cisternostomy for traumatic ASDH patients resulted in a somewhat improved but statistically nonsignificant outcome. Further extensive clinical trials are required to determine whether this approach should replace standard decompressive craniotomy in such cases.

In a Chinese journal of TBI[6] there was a case pertaining to a 35-year-old male individual who suffered severe TBI as a result of a road vehicle accident. He presented with ASDH, a GCS score of 6, fixed pupils, and absence of corneal response. Basal cisternostomy in conjunction with DC was executed, resulting in immediate brain relaxation. Postoperatively, the individual displayed notable progress, achieving a GCS score of 15 by the 6th day post-procedure. Subsequently, his condition continued to ameliorate, leading to his discharge on the 10th day post-surgery. The favorable outcome of this particular case implies that basal cisternostomy, through the act of opening the basal cisterns to atmospheric pressure and draining CSF, can represent a viable and efficacious approach in the treatment of TBI, potentially resulting in unforeseen positive recovery.

An investigation was held by Aline Lariessy Campos Paiva et al[7] in the year 2020. The primary objective of this investigation was to delineate the methodology, indications, and constraints of cisternostomy while drawing parallels with DC. TBI stands as a significant contributor to global mortality rates. Despite limited progress in recent years, there have been notable advancements in surgical strategies aimed at enhancing patient outcomes. Microsurgical cistern-ostomy, a well-established procedure in vascular and skull base surgery, has recently emerged as a viable option due to its reduced costs and morbidity when compared to DC for individuals with diffuse TBI. A prospective investigation is presently underway subsequent to the requisite approval from the local ethics research committee overseeing human subjects. Following the application of predetermined inclusion and exclusion criteria, patients undergo microsurgical cisternostomy, with assessments conducted on pre- and postoperative neurological status alongside brain computed tomography (CT) scans. Additionally, a comprehensive analysis encompassing diffuse TBI, DC, and cisternostomy as therapeutic interventions is undertaken. Among the patients subjected to cisternostomy post-TBI, two individuals exhibited ASDH and significant midline shift upon initial CT evaluation. Surgical intervention was sanctioned following family consent through the completion of informed consent forms. Subsequent to the procedure, both the patients exhibited favorable recovery trajectories and demonstrated satisfactory outcomes in follow-up brain CT scans, obviating the necessity for further surgical interventions post initial cisternostomy. Hence, cisternostomy emerges as a suitable therapeutic modality for a specific cohort of individuals grappling with diffuse TBI, presenting itself as a viable substitute to DC owing to its cost-effectiveness and reduced morbidity, underpinned by the execution of a singular neurosurgical intervention. Ongoing prospective research endeavors are underway to afford a more comprehensive assessment, with these initial cases laying the foundation for this novel protocol.

On further reviewing the literature of cisternostomy and its effectiveness in TBI, a prospective observational study was conducted at a single tertiary center by Ramesh Chandra Vemula et al[8] in the year 2022 which focused on management of the secondary brain injury in TBI patients. The study aimed to enlighten on the concept that since the brain and cisterns communicate, if there is pressure developing in any of these two compartments due to any cause, the pressure can be reduced by opening up the cisterns to the atmospheric pressure. In the study evaluating patients with TBI, a total of 25 patients underwent cisternostomy with intraoperative ICP monitoring. They were categorized into mild, moderate, and severe head injury groups based on GCS score. The patients were further classified into four groups based on age. The mortality rate observed in the study was 32%. At the 3-month follow-up, 48% of the patients showed good recovery with a GOS score of 4 and 5. The mean ICP after cisternostomy was recorded as $6.36 \pm 1.91$ mmHg. Importantly, there was a significant decrease in ICP after cisternostomy, indicating a positive impact of the procedure on ICP management in TBI patients.

A prospective longitudinal study was conducted on patients who underwent surgery between the year 2021 and 2022 by M.J. Encarnacion Ramirez et al[9] and based on the provided study data, it can be concluded that there were 30 patients included in the study, with 21 men and 9 women meeting the inclusion criteria. Among them, 80% underwent DC combined with cisternostomy, while 20% underwent cisternostomy alone. The initial GCS score at admission ranged from 4 to 8 points, with an average score of 5.9. The overall mortality and morbidity rates were 13.3 and 20%, respectively. The mortality rates were 12.5 and 16.7% in the DC + cisternostomy group and cisternostomy alone group, respectively. There was no statistically significant difference between the two groups in terms of mortality, morbidity, and favorable outcomes at 2 weeks, 3 months, and 6 months. Hence, based on the preliminary multi-center study findings, patients who underwent DC + cisternostomy or cisternostomy alone showed favorable clinical outcomes in both early and long-term follow-up. However, to establish the effectiveness of cisternostomy in the management of TBI, larger multi-center randomized trials are required.

Agung Bagus Sista Satyarsa et al[10] did a systematic review and meta-analysis on "The effectivity and safety of cisternostomy and decompressive craniectomy as management of brain trauma," focusing on proving that cisternostomy can be used as adjuvant management strategy for TBI, and the goal was also to address the lack of documentation regarding the use of cisternostomy in TBI management. The search was conducted using the

PubMed, Cochrane library, and Medline databases, focusing on publications in English within the last 10 years until June 2022. The evidence levels of each study were assessed by the Oxford Center for Evidence-Based Medicine. Data analysis was performed using RevMan version 5.3. Based on the information provided, the meta-analysis included four studies, consisting of two randomized controlled trials (RCTs) and two observational studies. The total number of patients included in the analysis was 1000, with 596 undergoing cisternostomies and 404 undergoing decompressive craniectomies. Key findings from the meta-analysis are as follows: (1) Mean GOS at 6 weeks: 0.93 (I2: 52%; 95%CI: 0.70 to 1.17; $p < 0.01$); (2) decrease in ICP post-operation: −3.20 mmHg (I2: 97%; 95%CI: −3.84 to −2.56; $p < 0.01$); (3) duration of ICU stay: −2.37 days (I2: 37%; 95%CI: −4.54 to −0.21; $p < 0.03$); (4) mortality rate: 0.51 (I2: 21%; 95%CI: 0.42 to 0.63; $p < 0.01$). The conclusion drawn from the meta-analysis is that cisternostomy is a beneficial procedure in TBI cases, resulting in improved survival rates and better clinical outcomes. The hope is that future studies will further investigate the role of cisternostomy in TBI patients.

A case report which was reported in April 2023 by Akram M. Eraky et al[11] stated that in a TBI-related delayed and prolonged elevation of ICP, cisternostomy is to be considered the treatment of option. Increased ICP can lead to brain herniation and reduced cerebral blood perfusion, causing ischemia. Recent studies have shown that cisternostomy with DC may offer better outcomes compared to DC alone for TBI patients. This improvement could be attributed to the understanding that cisternal CSF communicates with cerebral interstitial fluid (IF) through Virchow-Robin spaces. By opening cisterns to atmospheric pressure, IF drainage may be induced, resulting in decreased ICP. In a 55-year-old man who suffered subdural hematomas, hemorrhagic contusions, and subarachnoid hemorrhage from a fall off a moving truck, refractory ICP elevation was observed despite various interventions. Although initial treatments like increased sedation, paralysis, cooling, saline, mannitol, and DC were attempted, lumbar drain (LD) placement provided beneficial results. However, the LD malfunctioned multiple times, leading to increased ventricular size and elevated ICP with each occurrence. Subsequently, the patient underwent cisternostomy and lamina terminalis fenestration, which successfully prevented further ICP elevations during the 1-month follow-up. Hence, this case highlights cisternostomy as a promising surgical option for managing prolonged ICP elevation in TBI patients.

In conclusion, basal cisternostomy emerges as an efficacious intervention for patients with TBI, offering improved outcomes and potentially obviating the need for blanket decompressive craniectomy procedures and their associated risks.

## References

1. Cherian I, Beltran M, Landi A, Alafaci C, Torregrossa F, Grasso G. Introducing the concept of "CSF-shift edema" in traumatic brain injury. J Neurosci Res 2018;96(4):744–752

2. Cherian I, Yi G, Munakomi S. Cisternostomy: replacing the age old decompressive hemicraniectomy? Asian J Neurosurg 2013;8(3):132–138

3. Masoudi MS, Rezaee E, Hakiminejad H, Tavakoli M, Sadeghpoor T. Cisternostomy for management of intracranial hypertension in severe traumatic brain injury; case report and literature review. Bull Emerg Trauma 2016;4(3):161–164

4. Youssef O, Ali TM, Anbar K, El-Shahawy O, Enayet A. Value of adding cisternostomy to decompressive hemicraniectomy in the management of traumatic acute subdural hematoma patients. Open Access Maced J Med Sci 2020;8:1014–1022

5. Parthiban JKBC, Sundaramahalingam S, Rao JB, et al. Basal cisternostomy—a microsurgical cerebro spinal fluid let out

procedure and treatment option in the management of traumatic brain injury. Analysis of 40 consecutive head injury patients operated with and without bone flap replacement following cisternostomy in a tertiary care centre in India. Neurol India 2021;69(2):328–333

6. Encarnacion Ramirez MJ, Barrientos Castillo RE, Vorobiev A, Kiselev N, Aquino AA, Efe IE. Basal cisternostomy for traumatic brain injury: a case report of unexpected good recovery. English Edition. Chin J Traumatol 2022;25(5):302–305

7. Paiva ALC, Araujo JLV, Lovato RM, Veiga JCE. Microsurgical cisternostomy for treating critical patients with traumatic brain injury—an alternative therapeutic approach. Brazilian Neurosurgery 2020;39(3):155–160

8. Vemula RC, Prasad BCM, Banavath HN, Kale PKG, Krishna N MM, Gokanapudi S. Outcomes and predictors of outcome with cisternostomy in the management of traumatic brain injury—a prospective observational study at a tertiary centre. Indian J Neurotrauma 2022;19(2):78–83

9. Encarnacion Ramirez M, Baez IP, Marszal Mangbel' Mikorska H, et al. The role of cisternostomy in the management of severe traumatic brain injury: a triple-center study. Surgeries (Basel) 2023;4(2):283–292

10. Satyarsa ABS, Wardhana DPW, Brahmantya IBY, Rosyid RM, Maliawan S. The effectivity and safety of cisternostomy and decompressive craniectomy as management of brain trauma: a systematic review and meta-analysis. Indonesia Journal of Biomedical Science 2023;17(1):38–46

11. Eraky AM, Treffy R, Hedayat HS. Cisternostomy as a surgical treatment for traumatic brain injury-related prolonged and delayed intracranial pressure elevation: a case report. Cureus 2023;15(4):e37508

# 10 Future Perspectives of Cisternostomy

*Iype cherian and Kodeeswaran M.*

## Introduction

The Virchow-Robin spaces (VRS), also known as perivascular spaces, are cavities lined by pia mater which run alongside small arteries and arterioles as they pass from the subarachnoid space into the brain parenchyma. These spaces are essential for transporting cerebrospinal fluid (CSF) and metabolites, playing a significant role in the glymphatic system. VRS are not only important for normal brain function but also have clinical implications in various central nervous system disorders, such as neurodegenerative diseases and traumatic brain injuries (TBIs). Understanding the anatomy and function of VRS is crucial for diagnosing and treating these conditions effectively.

## Importance of Virchow-Robin Spaces in Various Neurological Conditions

VRS have significant implications in several neurological conditions and therapeutic approaches listed below:

- CSF shift edema in trauma: Following TBI, changes in CSF dynamics and VRS can lead to cerebral edema and increased intracranial pressure. Understanding these spaces is crucial for managing post-traumatic brain swelling and optimizing patient outcomes.

- Brain cooling and cleaning: Recent studies suggest that CSF flow through VRS helps clear metabolic waste from the brain, similar to a glymphatic system. Enhancing this process, possibly through therapeutic cooling techniques, could aid in neuroprotection and recovery after brain injury or neurodegenerative diseases.

- Neurodegenerative diseases: In conditions like Alzheimer's disease, impaired glymphatic function through VRS may contribute to the accumulation of amyloid-beta plaques and tau protein tangles. Targeting VRS pathways could offer new therapeutic avenues for slowing disease progression and enhancing clearance mechanisms.

# Possibilities of High-Grade Glioma Spreading through CSF and Virchow-Robin Spaces: Implications and Future Directions

High-grade gliomas (HGGs), such as glioblastoma multiforme (GBM), are highly aggressive brain tumors known for their rapid progression and poor prognosis. A comprehensive understanding of the mechanisms of dissemination via CSF and VRS is essential for developing effective treatments and improving patient outcomes.

## Spread Mechanisms of High-Grade Gliomas

High-grade gliomas are known for infiltrating surrounding brain tissue, making complete surgical resection challenging and often leading to recurrence. Besides direct infiltration into adjacent brain parenchyma, these tumors can disseminate through CSF pathways and exploit VRS which is described below.

## CSF Spread

Glioma cells can disseminate through the CSF, moving from the primary tumor site to distant areas in the brain and spinal cord. This dissemination can lead to leptomeningeal metastases, where tumor cells deposit along the meninges, resulting in secondary lesions. Recent studies indicate that glioma cells can travel via CSF pathways and establish themselves in the leptomeninges, contributing to disease progression and treatment resistance.

## Virchow-Robin Spaces (VRS)

VRS are perivascular spaces surrounding penetrating vessels from the subarachnoid space to the brain parenchyma. These spaces facilitate the transportation of immune cells, fluids, and potentially tumor cells within the brain. Glioma cells can migrate along VRS, infiltrating deeper brain regions, contributing to tumor progression, and presenting treatment challenges.

# Future Treatment Plans Targeting Virchow-Robin Spaces

Future research and therapeutic strategies may focus on leveraging VRS for targeted treatments:

- Enhanced drug delivery: Utilizing VRS for targeted drug delivery could improve the efficacy of chemotherapy or immunotherapy in treating gliomas. Nanoparticle-based carriers designed to traverse VRS and release therapeutic agents directly into tumor-invaded regions are under investigation.

- Modulation of CSF flow: Strategies to enhance CSF flow through VRS, such as pharmacological agents or mechanical interventions, could support brain cooling, enhance clearance mechanisms, and potentially mitigate neurodegenerative processes.
- Diagnostic and monitoring tools: Advancements in imaging techniques, including high-resolution MRI and dynamic contrast-enhanced MRI, may allow better visualization and monitoring of VRS integrity and function in various neurological disorders.

## Conclusion

Understanding the role of VRS in the spread of high-grade gliomas and its broader implications in neurological health is critical for developing innovative treatment strategies. Recent studies also suggest a potential link between VRS and the clearance of toxic waste products from the brain, highlighting avenues for further research into neurodegenerative diseases. Future research focusing on enhancing CSF dynamics, leveraging VRS for targeted therapies, and improving diagnostic tools holds promise in advancing the field and improving patient outcomes.

### Suggested Readings

Engelhardt B, Carare RO, Bechmann I, Flügel A, Laman JD, eller RO. Vascular, glial, and lymphatic immune gateways of he central nervous system. Acta Neuropathol 2016;132(3): 317–338

Hladky SB, Barrand MA. Mechanisms of fluid movement into, hrough and out of the brain: evaluation of the evidence. Fluids Barriers CNS 2014;11(1):26

Iliff JJ, Wang M, Liao Y, et al. A paravascular pathway facilitates CSF flow through the brain parenchyma and the clearance of interstitial solutes, including amyloid β. Sci Transl Med 2012;4(147):147ra111

Louis DN, Perry A, Reifenberger G, et al. The 2016 World Health Organization Classification of Tumors of the Central Nervous System: a summary. Acta Neuropathol 2016;131(6):803–820

Plog BA, Nedergaard M. The glymphatic system in central nervous system health and disease: past, present, and future. Annu Rev Pathol 2018;13:379–94

Taoka T, Masutani Y, Kawai H, et al. Evaluation of glymphatic system activity with the diffusion MR technique: diffusion tensor image analysis along the perivascular space (DTI-ALPS) in Alzheimer' disease cases. Jpn J Radiol 2017;35(4):172–78

# 11 | Cisternostomy: Complications and Its Management

*Pablo Villanueva and Iype Cherian*

## Introduction

Cisternostomy is a new and emerging surgical technique for head trauma which has proven to be a better alternative to decompressive hemicraniectomy. However, this is a complex procedure using skull base and vascular microsurgical principles and the chances for complications are higher compared to the rather simple, but defunct, decompressive hemicraniectomy.

During the execution of a surgical intervention, the operating surgeon must possess foreknowledge of potential complications in order to effectively anticipate and manage unforeseen circumstances. It is widely acknowledged that the complexity of a procedure directly correlates with the likelihood of additional complications arising. The causes of a complication can be categorized based on its underlying etiology: complications stemming from the pathology itself, those arising from technical challenges, and those resulting from accidental or unexpected events.

# Pathology "Per Se" Complication

The primary indication for performing a cisternostomy is the presence of severe brain edema. It is reasonable to anticipate challenges associated with this condition. Brain edema, through the addition of excess volume of fluid to the cerebral parenchyma (refer CSF shift edema in Chapter 4 and 9), exerts pressure on all the relevant structures. Consequently, blood vessels exhibit congestion, the gray matter loses its typical boundaries (resulting in visibility issues), and the white matter becomes fragile (displaying unstable surfaces) and nonelastic.

All these aforementioned circumstances contribute to the brain's susceptibility to hemorrhaging and render it rather challenging to manage. In certain cases, with markedly elevated intracranial pressure, brain spatula retraction of the lateral basifrontal lobes to reach the opticocarotid and the lateral carotid cisterns even following extensive initial decompression of the sphenoid ridge may be challenging.

In the subsequent brief passages, various scenarios will be illustrated, and each will be evaluated independently.

## Challenges Regarding Visibility

Upon opening the dura mater, one will encounter a tightly situated brain beneath. The identification of brain orientation and distinguishing features may prove to be a challenging task. The region known as Broca's area, demarcated by the boundaries of the pars triangularis, demands careful consideration, particularly on the left hemisphere. However, this becomes a formidable endeavor in cases of brain displacement when locating the sulci presents difficulties.

In instances where conventional techniques yield unsatisfactory results, it is important to take out all the basal bone including the lesser wing of sphenoid and shave off the optic roof as thin as possible in an extradural fashion. Failure to do so may exacerbate the existing visual obstructions, leading to complications in the near future.

**The following may be undertaken in order to alleviate this uncomfortable scenario:**

- It is imperative that every possible medical intervention is utilized to reduce the existing brain edema to the greatest extent achievable. This includes ensuring proper perfusion and ventilation, considering options such as hyperventilation and hypothermia, optimizing the acid–base status and ionic balance, and implementing active pharmacological treatments such as mannitol and 3% NaCl.

- In our perspective, a correct position of the head and an appropriately sized craniotomy are recommended. The size should typically facilitate adequate exposure (reaching the temporal base, providing entry to temporal and frontal poles, and ensuring full visibility of the sphenoidal ridge up to the anterior clinoidal process). This approach addresses the surgical approach issue effectively. Different countries or medical facilities have varying practices, with some opting for minimal bone flap sizes while others performing decompressive craniectomy simultaneously. Each scenario presents its own advantages and disadvantages.

- In order to achieve success during the surgical procedure, it is imperative to execute all necessary surgical techniques such as hematoma evacuation, contusion treatment, and bone fragments excision as indicated. However, **the most important part of the procedure is to remove the skull base as much as possible including the sphenoid ridge and shaving off the orbital roof in an extradural fashion.**

- If the previously mentioned approaches prove to be ineffective, the gradual application of frontal lobe retraction should be initiated until a significant anatomical structure like the olfactory nerve, optic nerve, or carotid is visualized. Subsequently, a minimal level of retraction surrounding the identified area must be conducted to ensure the continuity of the surgical intervention.

- During the cisternostomy procedure, the frontal lobes typically protrude prominently. Delicate retraction maneuvers combined with slow movements are essential to reach the optic nerve and detach the arachnoid of the optic nerve from the frontal lobe arachnoid thereby opening the cisterns. Proficiency in maintaining focus and adjusting the viewing angle with the aid of visual enhancement tools such as a microscope or exoscope is crucial.

- Upon identification of critical structures such as the carotid artery or optic nerve, it is imperative to preserve these landmarks at all costs. Failure to reach this milestone may result in irreparable parenchymal damage or the need for extensive resection. Subsequently, the opening of the carotid cistern through the opto-carotid triangle window is a pivotal maneuver to reduce intracranial pressure intraoperatively and achieve the desired surgical outcome. This action facilitates the drainage of cerebrospinal fluid and edematous content from the cistern, thereby causing relaxation of the brain.

## Unstable Surfaces

Accessing the anterior skull base is a challenging task even under optimal circumstances; therefore, performing this in unfavorable conditions such as swelling, bleeding, or instability requires thorough preparation, expertise, knowledge, and innovative techniques.

Various solutions may need to be considered depending on the underlying cause of the issue. Adequate bone drilling is of paramount importance. If a parenchymal surface is bleeding or fails to respond to gentle retraction, leading to bulging in the line of sight, further retraction can be done in the basifrontal area leading to the optic nerve first, and this would lead usually to an egress of blood and CSF which will result in a "breathing space" during which time the other cisternal openings and washing out the blood can be initiated.

In such instances, several strategies can be employed to enhance retraction on unstable surfaces. Options include switching to a wider or narrower retractor based on the condition of the surface—a narrower retractor may be preferred for undamaged surfaces, while a wider one could be more suitable for contused or compromised brain tissue. Additionally, the application of thin silicone membranes on the retractor surface or the utilization of tubular retractors commonly used in endoscopic procedures may offer alternative solutions. Other potential strategies include placing wet gauze on the surface, maintaining continuous irrigation, and using Surgicel on compromised areas, among others. These suggestions are intended to stimulate creative thinking and aid in developing personalized solutions.

Instances of trauma-induced alterations also merit attention: the presence of a craniofacial injury may lead to significant disruptions in the anterior skull base. A meticulous preoperative assessment through CT scanning plays a crucial role in averting serious errors when approaching the central cisterns.

# Technical Complications

Technical complications refer to challenges arising in complex situations, leading to changes in anatomical structures and standard procedures.

## Mistakes Related to the Handling of Microscopes/ Exoscopes

- There is only one piece of advice on this subject matter: individuals lacking proficiency in managing and optimizing the visual aid system should abstain from performing a cisternostomy procedure.
- This specific scenario encompasses numerous unforeseen circumstances and anatomical alterations. The presence of such variability, coupled with additional technical challenges in achieving adequate visualization, may result in hazards.

## Safe Unlocking

- The term "safe unlocking" (orbitomeningeal band) refers to a crucial procedure that enables the brain to be mobile during the surgeon's approach to the opto-carotid triangle.
- The orbitomeningeal band is a consistently positioned thickened layer of meningeal tissue located above the superior margin of the superior orbital fissure. Dissecting it from the temporal pole dura ensures the preservation of the cavernous sinus covering adjacent to it, facilitating access from the lateral to medial direction toward the anterior clinoid process.
- Executing this procedure correctly ensures that the subsequent stages of the surgery are merely a matter of time. Beneath the clinoid process lie significant structures that grant entry to the carotid cistern, followed by

the interpeduncular cistern, Liliequist membrane, and ultimately, the prepontine cistern, which serves as the final destination for the drainage tip.

- Clinoidectomy is a matter of choice; however, in very tight brains the authors prefer to do the extradural clinoidectomy. This opens up the access to opticocarotid cisterns. Basal dural opening is another important procedure and after this, the retraction to lead to the optic nerve along the lateral basifrontal lobe is important.

## Dissection at Deep Stages

- Microsurgical expertise will be essential in this context. Targeting arachnoid membranes in a brain affected by trauma poses challenges, given the presence of bleeding and the visual and retraction difficulties previously discussed.
- Regular irrigation with cold saline is imperative, not only to enhance dissection precision but also to achieve a "cooling and refreshing" effect to reduce the potential consequences of edema.

## Handling of Contused Lobes

- Cerebral contusions are a common coexisting injury seen in cases of severe diffuse edema. The frontal and temporal lobes are the most commonly impacted regions, often as a result of direct or indirect trauma forces experienced during the initial injury event.
- Characterized by a fragile mass of brain tissue with a necrotic core, contusions exhibit vessel fragility and cellular edema due to dysfunction of cerebral membranes within the affected area.
- Surgical intervention, such as partial or complete removal of the contused tissue, may be necessary to

prevent inflammation and create space for further cisternal exploration. Essential to the success of this procedure is the ability to effectively control bleeding during the resection process. Avoiding bipolar forceps and just using a surgical with a gelfoam and cotton patty placed over it is the best way of dealing with these contusions. When they are large enough, usage of a cortical incision and letting them out with gentle suction can help with regional cerebral perfusion pressure in the postoperative course.

## Handling of Subdural and Cisternal Hemorrhages

Subdural and cisternal hemorrhages management involves addressing the temporal relationship between the traumatic event and the initiation of cranial surgery, resulting in the presence of delicate yet cohesive materials within the subdural or cisternal compartments. Merely employing washing techniques may prove insufficient, necessitating meticulous dissection, suction, and occasionally hemostasis using bipolar forceps within the affected area.

# Non-anticipated Occurrences

## Recognition of Profuse Bleeding (in Dural Sinus, Carotid Tearing)

- Decompression seen in cisternostomy may sometimes lead to unmasking of a sinus injury that was present and severe bleeding.
- It might become essential to pack a dural sinus or pack the bleeding edges with fibrillar Surgicel and to raise the head in these circumstances. Despite an unfavorable prognosis, this particular maneuver becomes indispensable for the completion of the surgical intervention.

## Damaging of Noble Structure

- Noble structures are prone to damage during dissection or retraction. The carotid artery, though visible and pliant, is not commonly damaged. Conversely, the optic nerve may exhibit particular vulnerability to manipulation, traction, and compression.
- Assessing the pupils before and during the procedure serves as a valuable metric in cases of rough manipulation or detected traumatic compression. The initial step involves releasing the noble structure, followed by resuming cisternal dissection.
- The opto-carotid triangle likely serves as the primary landmark in the procedure. Delicate handling of these structures is essential and necessitates training. Subsequent stages such as cisternal dissection, identification of elements, and Liliequist opening demand similar or even higher levels of skill and caution. This phase of the surgery requires a deliberate approach to ensure safety, accuracy, and efficiency, without haste. "आरामसे—aaraamase [gently, easy]" the author's mentor, Dr. Cherian would always remind him, while learning about cisternostomy at Krishna Vishwa Vidyapeeth in Karad, upon sighting the carotid and optic nerve.

## The Drainage Catheter

- Recognition of cisterns relies on the identification of components situated within the confines of the area. Boundary visibility is hindered by both dissection and compression, making it imperative to accurately reach the tip of the basilar artery to ensure proper placement of the drainage catheter into the prepontine space between the pons and the clivus.

- Upon identification of the element and successful access to the prepontine space, the drainage catheter must be positioned accordingly.
- It is considered a prudent practice for the assistant to secure the drainage catheter in place and sustain a continuous flow of irrigation through it. The assistant should verify the catheter's position by recognizing specific markers on its surface to prevent any inadvertent movement until it is securely fixed at the opposite end.
- During the surgeon's commencement of revision, hemostasis assessment, and final cleansing of the cavity, it is recommended to manually secure the catheter's position against a prominent anatomical landmark. This aspect is crucial in the surgical procedure and carries a significant responsibility for the assistant.
- In addition to holding the catheter steady, it is essential to ensure its stability until the conclusion of the surgery and its fixation onto the skin. Furthermore, continuous irrigation and letting out should be sustained to guarantee the catheter's patency.
- Should any issues arise during these procedures, the assistant should promptly communicate, conduct a thorough inspection of the drainage system, and refrain from proceeding with the closure until the placement and fixation of the drainage catheter are definitively confirmed.

## The Patient's Condition Was Precarious Prior to Achieving the Surgical Objective

- Facing an unstable patient prior to achieving the surgical objective is the ultimate fear for each trauma surgeon. The key to averting this dire scenario lies in meticulous preoperative preparations aimed at not only achieving optimal hemodynamic and respiratory stability but also ensuring readiness to address edema and its repercussions throughout the surgical intervention.

- According to the perspective of authors, once advancements in technique are made and the procedure can be executed with enhanced safety measures, anesthetists assume a pivotal role in supporting the operator. It is very important to maintain the blood pressure from the emergency department to the dural opening and decompression as the failure of this may be the single most important reason for failure. Blood loss correction, fluid correction, correction of acidosis, electrolytes etc. are other importance steps to ensure the success of a cisternostomy procedure.

- Usage of vasopressors should be limited and should be only done for a short time when a fluid challenge fails to maintain adequate blood pressure. This is another important lesson.

## Conclusion

Surgical procedures inherently incorporate an element of artistry. This is especially evident in the context of trauma, where unpredictability prevails, underscoring the importance of gleaning insights from seasoned experts. The adeptness of these individuals, when appropriately harnessed and shared as counsel, stands as a cornerstone for ensuring the safety and success of a procedure.

While cisternostomy represents a novel approach, thorough anatomical comprehension and systematic instruction have the potential to elevate it to the status of a benchmark technique. This transformation could prove pivotal in addressing the current prevalent crisis of brain trauma and its profound impact on the younger demographic.

# Index

# The fundamental, one-stop global resource for neurosurgical practice in updated 10th edition

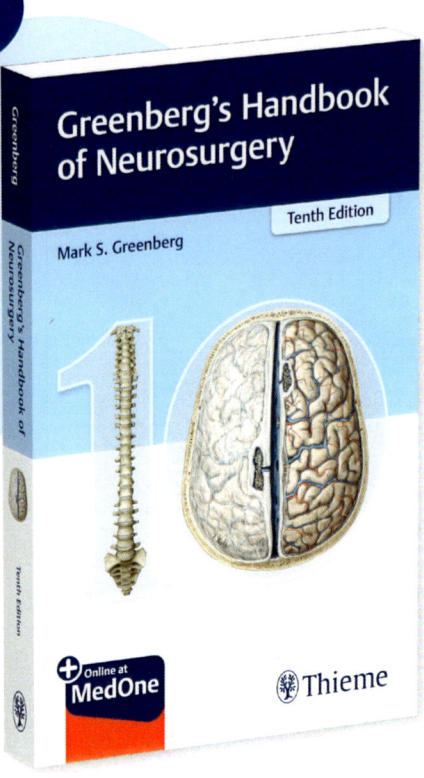

The comprehensive, conveniently compact book provides detailed, high-value, and actionable information that can be quickly accessed to enhance patient management, thereby eliminating the need to wade through superfluous material. It is also a perfect study companion for board examination and preparation for the maintenance of certification.

## Key Highlights

- Updated classification and diagnostic criteria of central and peripheral nervous system tumors, based on the most recent WHO classifications
- Reworking of numerous sections (including current concepts in pseudotumor cerebri, seizure classification...)
- Addition of new chapters (including idiopathic scoliosis, LOVA and tuberculosis of the CNS)
- Current principles of nonsurgical and surgical management, including risk factors, indications, diagnostics, prognoses, contraindications, and differential diagnoses
- Nearly 500 figures, including new summary flow charts, illustrations, and simplified diagrams for early learners, enhance understanding of material discussed in the text and, as always, thousands of references!

This print book includes complimentary access to a digital copy on https://medone.thieme.com.

Publisher's Note: Products purchased from Third Party sellers are not guaranteed by the publisher for quality, authenticity, or access to any online entitlements included with the product.

ISBN : 9781684205042  |  Binding : Paperback
Edition :10th  |  Date : May 2023
Pages :1800  |  Illustrations : 250

**SCAN THE QR CODE
TO ORDER TODAY**

shop.thieme.in

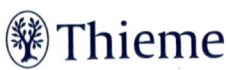